The Bipolar Disorder Workbook

THE
Bipolar
Disorder
WORKBOOK

Powerful Tools & Practical Resources for
BIPOLAR II AND CYCLOTHYMIA

PETER FORSTER, MD
with Gina Gregory, LCSW

ALTHEA
PRESS

This book is dedicated to my wife, Kelli Craft, who passed away unexpectedly after the book was written. She was a strong supporter of the project and would be so happy to think of the help that it will offer to those who wrestle with bipolar. —P.F.

Cover Design: William D. Mack
Interior Design: Meg Woodcheke
Editor: Camille Hayes
Production Editor: Erum Khan

ISBN: Print 978-1-64152-063-8 | eBook 978-1-64152-064-5

CONTENTS

INTRODUCTION

OUR EXPERIENCE WORKING TOGETHER in a multidisciplinary clinic that specializes in treating people with bipolar disorder and unipolar depression inspired us to write this book. We find that most people confronting the challenges of bipolar disorder can build good lives: lives that matter and that reward the people living them. This doesn't mean we underestimate the obstacles people who are wrestling with bipolar face; on the contrary, we recognize their unique strengths.

Many of our patients have used the periods of energy and creativity associated with bipolar to produce brilliant apps, works of art, architectural designs, start-up plans, and much more. The key to their success is being able to effectively manage their moods and create a work environment that supports these moments of inspiration, while allowing for periods of reduced productivity as well. With effort and some tenacity, you, too, can live a full and rewarding life with bipolar disorder.

Our optimism is also based in our knowledge of the developing scientific understanding of what causes bipolar and cyclothymia and how to minimize the negative effects of these conditions. For instance, recently there has been an explosion of knowledge about how the internal clock that regulates sleep and wakefulness affects mood stability. The following example from our practice illustrates how an insight like this—and other techniques you'll find in this workbook—can transform a life that might feel as though it were hurtling toward catastrophe.

Richard was a man in the midst of a brutal divorce (which would separate him from the son he loved), living with a brilliant but unstable journalist and supervising one of the largest and most controversial building projects in the San Francisco Bay Area at the time. He was smart, charismatic, and accomplished in his field, but his life was such a wreck that when we first met him, he was seriously contemplating suicide.

We were quickly able to identify the pattern of periods of deep depression alternating with periods of unusual energy and accomplishment (as well as risk-taking) that often marks the creative individual with bipolar II. This allowed us to make better choices for which medications to treat his depression and also opened a productive discussion of the "problem" of his hypomania. His previous psychiatrist had assumed that treating his depression was enough, but we could see quite clearly that what led to his depressions was his fascination with the excitement of his hypomanic periods. He was like a moth drawn to the light. Richard was aware that his crashes often came after periods of inadequate sleep and a crazy work schedule of dawn-to-midnight meetings and planning sessions, but he was unable to moderate his behavior.

When working on previous projects, he always had to have a colleague who could make up for some of the excesses of his hypomanic periods, patch things up with those he offended, and fill in when he was depressed. Over time we were able to show him how a combination of better sleep habits, regular exercise, less drinking (alcohol was part of what made his sleep so poor during hypomanic periods), mindfulness meditation, and increased awareness and acceptance of both the strengths and weaknesses of his bipolar allowed him to function more steadily. Importantly, Richard also learned that this greater stability didn't cause him to lose the creative genius that he brought to his work.

With greater mood stability, he was also able to patch up the chaos of his personal life. Eventually he resolved the conflict with his ex-wife and resumed his relationship with his beloved son. And he moved from the turbulence of his affair with the unstable journalist to a relationship with a dear woman who was able to support his new way of life. This tremendous life growth all began with a relatively simple sleep intervention and expanded from there.

Over the years, it has been our privilege to work with people with bipolar and cyclothymia, helping them reshape their lives for the better. In our clinic, we use the same kinds of exercises and interventions that are in this workbook, and we know they work. Time and again, we've seen people successfully learn to manage their bipolar II or cyclothymia. Transforming a life takes time, but now that you have this workbook in your hands, you, too, can begin to relaunch your life. You're holding the right tool.

HOW TO USE THIS BOOK

THIS BOOK HAS BEEN WRITTEN IN A PARTICULAR ORDER. The ideas, skills, and techniques in each chapter build on the ones before, so we strongly recommend that you work through the book in order, chapter by chapter. However, there's no need to rush through the book. In fact, it may make sense to take the chapters at a relatively slow pace, depending on your schedule.

Our experience in leading groups of people with bipolar through a somewhat similar program suggests that one chapter a week is a good pace for many. But as you work through the exercises, if you want or need to take a break for whatever reason, that's fine, too. Because you may want to practice these exercises more than once, it's a good idea to make some copies of them before filling them out in the workbook.

We begin by looking at the idea of diagnosis. Diagnosis in psychiatry is controversial for many reasons. It oversimplifies issues, reduces personal experiences to symptoms, and is not as reliable as we would like. But diagnosis does allow us to compare experiences and find patterns that can guide effective change, which is why we begin this book by looking at it in depth.

As we take you through a discussion of the symptoms of bipolar II and cyclothymia, you will see whether, and how, this workbook applies to your unique life situation.

After we explore diagnosis, we review some effective therapies for bipolar. Although not an exhaustive list, it includes almost all the tools we routinely use in our clinic. We focus on therapeutic tools drawn from Cognitive Behavioral Therapy (CBT) and Acceptance and Commitment Therapy (ACT). These ideas, as well as ones from Interpersonal and Social Rhythm Therapy (IPSRT) and Cognitive Behavioral Analysis System of Psychotherapy (CBASP), are the basis for most of the exercises in this workbook.

Each of you will pick up this workbook and begin using it at a different point in your life and with different experiences of coping with your symptoms. Some may know relatively little about the condition, while others may have a lot of knowledge and experience. In part 1, before we jump into the heart of the workbook, we help you assess where you are now, at the beginning of this journey.

Part 2 focuses on energized states (for example, hypomania and mixed-mood episodes). During these periods, it's common to experience a greater sense of confidence in your ability to do things, which can be exciting but may also be risky if the feelings are unrealistic. How can you tell when having a great day is something to be concerned about? We help you find answers to this question. At other times, energized states may present with symptoms of agitation and irritability. In this book, you will learn techniques for coping with extreme mood states such as these.

Part 3 will help you cope with depression, which is often the most disabling symptom of bipolar. We talk about the various ways depression can affect your life, and we show you how relatively small changes in daily activity can help prevent, shorten, and minimize depressive symptoms.

Next, we show you how to create a personal plan for dealing with the risky behaviors that can be associated with depression, hypomania, or mixed-mood states.

Finally, we talk about the importance of having a team, or support network, to help you cope with bipolar II and cyclothymia more effectively. We guide you through the process of creating and sustaining an effective team, and give you tools to help you resolve conflicts that can sabotage relationships.

Being physically strong and healthy is of great importance to living well with bipolar II or cyclothymia. Throughout the workbook, you'll see Whole-Health Strategy sidebars that give you tips and concrete ways to improve your physical well-being.

In the final chapter, we talk about how to prioritize these tools: which ones to make a regular part of your life and which ones to save for future use. By the time you reach the end of this workbook, you will have a set of tools and a strategy in place that will help you create the kind of life you want and deserve.

PART ONE

Definitions & Treatments

In this section of the workbook,, we review the diagnoses covered in this workbook (bipolar II, cyclothymia, and other bipolar disorders). We discuss the mood states that define them, including hypomania (mild mania) and depression, as well as how they differ from bipolar I (which is not a focus for this workbook). You'll find an overview of different treatment approaches for these conditions, focusing particularly on non-medication treatments, and ways you can benefit from these treatments, even if you aren't able to find a clinician who is a bipolar expert. Make copies of the exercises before filling them out in the workbook so you can have some on hand for later practice.

CHAPTER ONE

Understanding Bipolar II Disorder & Cyclothymia

THIS CHAPTER INTRODUCES THE KEY FEATURES of bipolar II, cyclothymia, and other bipolar disorders—what we call the "bipolar spectrum disorders"—and how these conditions differ from bipolar I, the most easily recognized and diagnosed form of bipolar.

Even though the concepts of hypomania and bipolar II have been recognized for the last 35 years in the *Diagnostic and Statistical Manual of Mental Disorders (DSM)*, bipolar spectrum disorders are often misunderstood. It's surprising how often we hear other mental health professionals express the belief that someone "can't really be bipolar" because they've never experienced a dramatic manic episode.

A nearly tragic example of this misunderstanding was a young woman—we'll call her Carrie—we saw more than 10 years ago. Although bright and charming, she often made impulsive decisions that turned out badly. She was in therapy with a well-respected Jungian analyst. Despite the analyst's wisdom, he had one flaw: He didn't know what he didn't know; that is, he didn't know where his expertise stopped. The analyst became convinced he could "understand" all of Carrie's impulsive decisions based on his Jungian view of the psyche. We saw Carrie at her mother's request for a second opinion. It seemed clear to us that Carrie had a bipolar mood disorder, for which we strongly recommended treatment with lithium. She initially had a positive response to the medication but also experienced annoying side effects.

At this point, Carrie's analyst stepped in with a recommendation that she focus on her treatment with him, so she stopped treatment with our mood disorder clinic. We were so concerned that we arranged to meet with the analyst to explain our diagnosis, but he was not convinced. Two years later, Carrie nearly died in a serious suicide attempt associated with a mixed episode of hypomanic and depressed symptoms. Fortunately, she recognized that the treatment she was receiving was inadequate, and she returned to our clinic. With appropriate care, her functioning, outlook, and life satisfaction improved greatly over time. This is just one example of the ways in which a thorough understanding of the bipolar spectrum is critically important to effective treatment.

Familiarize Yourself with Your Diagnosis

If you have been recently diagnosed with bipolar disorder or cyclothymia, you may have had an opportunity to talk about some of the key concepts and symptoms that define these conditions. However, because the concepts can be complicated, and because being told you have some form of bipolar can be an emotionally charged experience, it's not uncommon to find that people who've been dealing with symptoms of bipolar for years still don't fully understand some of the basic concepts. Our first step in this program is to ensure that you have the knowledge you need in order to take on the challenge of managing your symptoms.

Mood disorders are divided into two categories:

1. Those that involve only experiencing either a "normal" mood or symptoms of depression, which are diagnosed as depressive disorders (for example, major depression or dysthymia)
2. Those that involve experiencing depression and an energized or activated state (hypomania, mania, or mixed symptoms of mania and depression), which are considered bipolar disorders

This workbook focuses on two kinds of bipolar disorder that are often misunderstood and misdiagnosed because they are not associated with the most intensely energized states (mania): bipolar II, or cyclothymia. We will also briefly touch on a set of conditions known as "other specified bipolar disorder" and "unspecified bipolar disorder," which we will group together and call "other bipolar disorders."

BIPOLAR II

Bipolar II is diagnosed when someone has experienced at least one hypomanic (mildly manic) episode and one episode of major (or serious) depression. Although you'll find hypomania defined in greater detail on page 6, for now, it's enough to consider it a milder mania that's not associated with severe impairment (and may not be associated with any impairment at all!) and that may be quite short—lasting as little as four days, in some cases.

Something that often confuses even experienced mental health clinicians is that a person who has experienced *only one* hypomanic episode in a lifetime, and who has had many episodes of major depression, is still considered to have bipolar II. This is because people who have had one hypomanic episode are much more likely to experience another one at some point in the future—so their recommended treatment needs to consider both types of mood episodes.

For most people, the distinction between bipolar depression and major depression unrelated to bipolar works reasonably well, but obviously the importance of energized or hypomanic symptoms in the treatment of someone with bipolar depends on the severity and frequency of those symptoms.

Someone who had one episode of hypomania 20 years ago, after being treated with an antidepressant, and has since only experienced either normal moods or depressive episodes is not the same as someone who routinely cycles between hypomania and depression. Each person's treatment needs to reflect their individual pattern of symptoms.

CYCLOTHYMIA

"Cyclothymia" is a condition associated with numerous mildly energized episodes and mildly depressed episodes over the course of at least two years. Because they are significantly less severe, the energized episodes don't meet the criteria for a hypomanic or manic episode, and the depressed episodes don't meet the criteria for a major depressive episode. During the two-year period, the person must have been in either an energized or depressed period for more than half the time.

In some cases, cyclothymia may develop into bipolar I or II. But a significant number of people experience this pattern of alternating, mild mood episodes without developing more severe symptoms.

Symptoms

The primary symptoms of bipolar II disorder and cyclothymia are hypomania and depression. Your experiences with these symptoms—how often you have them and how severely they affect your life—will vary, but the following information will help you understand how mood cycles affect your life and what you can do about them.

HYPOMANIA

A hypomanic episode is a distinct and noticeable period with a persistently elated, joyful, or irritable mood and unusually increased activity or energy that lasts four days or longer. During that period, three of the following symptoms must be present:

- An unrealistic belief in your ability to do things (grandiosity)
- A decreased need for sleep
- Notably increased talkativeness
- Distractibility (being drawn to things that you wouldn't ordinarily notice)
- Increased activity (doing more at home, work, or school)
- Doing things that are risky (spending too much money, engaging in unusual sexual activity, taking on risky business investments, and so on)

A hypomanic episode is not associated with severe impairment or psychotic symptoms and shouldn't require hospitalization. The presence of any of those characteristics—impairment, psychosis, hospitalization—means that the episode is mania rather than hypomania.

To meet the diagnostic criteria for bipolar II, an episode of hypomania can't be due to a medical condition or the use of a medication or substance (for example, taking a stimulant or hallucinogen). There's a special note in the diagnostic criteria addressing the common issue of a hypomanic episode associated with taking an antidepressant. If the symptoms last only as long as the medication stays in your body, the episode isn't considered to be hypomania. However, an episode that's triggered by an antidepressant but persists after the medication has left your body is considered hypomania.

Think back on the last time you felt energized. Did you experience any of the symptoms we described? How long did the episode last? Did other people notice that your behavior was different? Answering these questions can be a step in determining whether you experienced hypomania or the closely related, but more extreme, symptoms of mania.

MANIA

Mania is a more dramatically energized state than hypomania. If you have ever had a manic episode, your diagnosis would be bipolar I disorder. To be considered mania, an episode must last at least seven days and be associated with either severe impairment (inability to work or perform self-care, alienation from friends and family) or psychotic symptoms (hallucinations, completely unrealistic beliefs, paranoia, or other delusions), or must require hospitalization.

Other than being more severe and lasting at least seven days, the symptoms of mania are the same as those for hypomania, although for most people, mania involves a more highly energized state. With that in mind, we've described some of the possible differences in the following Hypomania Symptoms exercise, which compares mania, hypomania, and a mildly energized state compatible with a cyclothymia diagnosis.

EXERCISE: HYPOMANIA SYMPTOMS

Think back to a time when you were particularly energetic, active, optimistic, or irritable. Which of these symptoms did you experience? It may help to get the perspective of someone who knows you well, since some of these symptoms might not be as obvious to you. Check all the boxes that apply.

SYMPTOM	SEVERE: MANIA	MODERATE: HYPOMANIA OR MANIA	MILD: CYCLOTHYMIA
Grandiosity	☐ Believing you can do anything	☒ Unrealistic sense of abilities	☒ Slightly optimistic view of capabilities
Reduced Sleep	☒ No sleep for several days	☒ Getting by on 4 to 5 hours of sleep	☒ Sleeping an hour or 2 fewer per day
Talkativeness	☒ Can't stop talking, texting, phoning; people are annoyed	☒ More talkative; talking to people you wouldn't usually talk to	☒ Longer than usual e-mails, more texting than normal, a little talkative
Distractibility	☒ Can't focus on anything for more than a few minutes; constantly distracted	☒ Noticing things that you wouldn't usually notice; colors brighter; smells richer; difficulty reading for long	☐ Enjoying the world of senses more, but able to focus when necessary
Increased Activity	☒ Nonstop activity	☒ Significantly increased activity, noticeable to others	☐ Slightly more active but not worrisome to others
Risky Behavior	☒ Clearly risky behavior, e.g., sexual affairs, spending money, or driving recklessly	☒ Somewhat risky behavior, e.g., spending too much money, unusual sexual activity	☒ More interest in sex; spending somewhat more money

As with hypomania, manic symptoms don't meet the criteria for bipolar I if they are caused by a medical condition, a medication, or substance use. But, as with hypomania, an episode of mania that's triggered by medication or substance use that lasts beyond the time the substance is present in your bloodstream does meet the criteria for bipolar I.

Distinguishing between hypomanic or manic symptoms caused by a medical condition, medication, or substance and ones merely triggered by such a condition is extremely tricky and beyond the scope of this workbook. If you have any questions about this, consult with a psychiatrist or psychologist who has expertise in treating and diagnosing bipolar disorders.

DEPRESSION

Generally, depression is a state that's the opposite of mania or hypomania: It's associated with decreased energy, lack of motivation, sadness, and the like. Later in this chapter, we'll talk about the special case of mixed symptoms (periods associated with increased energy but a depressive mood) and depressive episodes that may be associated with symptoms that can occur in mania or hypomania (such as agitation and insomnia). But for now, let's focus on the more typical experience of depressive symptoms.

DEPRESSION CHECKLIST

A major depressive episode is a period of at least two weeks during which you experience five or more of the following symptoms. To learn more about your experiences of depression, complete the short self-assessment below. Place a check next to a symptom if you have experienced it in the past.

- ☑ A depressed, sad, empty, hopeless, or tearful mood during most of the day and nearly every day for two weeks

- ☑ Markedly decreased interest or enjoyment in all or almost all activities during most of the day and nearly every day for two weeks

- ☑ Loss of more than 5 percent of body weight in a month without dieting, or a significant decrease in appetite nearly every day for two weeks

- ☑ Gain of more than 5 percent of body weight in a month, or a significant increase in appetite nearly every day for two weeks

- ☑ Insomnia (reduced sleep without decreased need for sleep) nearly every day for two weeks

- ☑ Hypersomnia (significantly increased sleep) nearly every day for two weeks

- ☑ Noticeable (to others) agitation nearly every day for two weeks

- ☑ Noticeable (to others) reduced movement nearly every day for two weeks

☑ Fatigue, tiredness, or reduced energy nearly every day for two weeks

☑ Feeling worthless or excessively guilty nearly every day for two weeks

☑ Reduced ability to think, concentrate, or make routine decisions nearly every day for two weeks

☑ Repeated thoughts of death or suicide, or a suicide attempt or plan to commit suicide

EXERCISE: DEPRESSION TYPES

People with depression may experience more than one type of depression. Is this true for you? Do you sometimes have depression associated with weight loss and decreased appetite, but other times experience an increased appetite? Do you sometimes have agitated and anxious or irritable depression and then, at other times, have depression associated with increased sleep and reduced energy? Think about the types of symptoms you usually experience and describe them here.

Extreme difficulty in reading and concentrating. Focused more on death. Worrying about it more often. Feeling extremely tired and not wanting to wake up in the morning. Sleeping way more than usual. Loss of interest in things usually interested in.

MIXED EPISODES

One of the significant changes in our understanding of mood episodes involves increasing recognition that the description of hypomanic, manic, and depressive episodes oversimplifies many people's experience of bipolar. The latest _Diagnostic and Statistical Manual of Mental Disorders_ (_DSM-5_) contains much greater acknowledgment of "mixed episodes": mood episodes associated with symptoms of hypomania or mania and symptoms of depression. These episodes are considered hypomanic, manic, or depressive based on the predominant symptoms and are then described as having "mixed features," to highlight the presence of symptoms usually unassociated with the primary mood state.

As an example, a hypomanic episode with mixed features might be feelings of hopelessness or despair and increased talkativeness and energy—things that we don't typically associate with depression. Such a mixed episode might include cynical and pessimistic thoughts *along with* agitation and impulsive decision-making.

Have you ever experienced mixed symptoms? These states can be particularly distressing and are potentially dangerous because the combination of hopelessness and increased energy is even more likely to lead to self-destructive acts than pure depression.

WHAT TO DO IF YOU'RE HAVING SUICIDAL OR SELF-HARMING THOUGHTS

If you're currently thinking about suicide or about harming yourself, or if you find yourself preoccupied with death or wishing for death, please take these thoughts seriously. Such thoughts are a sign that the stresses you face are greater than your coping resources. The need for help that they represent must be attended to.

- **Talk to someone now.** The National Suicide Prevention Lifeline (1-800-273-8255) is available 24 hours a day, seven days a week, and is free to anyone in the United States.

- **Let someone know.** One of the terrible things that sometimes happens when we have suicidal thoughts is that we withdraw from the very people who could support us. Even though it may be hard, this is a time when it's essential to share our pain. Let someone know you've been feeling overwhelmed, even if you can't let them know how overwhelmed.

Beginning conversations with those who love you is important.

- **Get professional help.** If you are in treatment with a mental health professional, let them know about your suicidal thoughts. Recognize that these thoughts are a sign that you need more help. If you are not in treatment, now is a good time to reach out for help.

- **Call 911 or go to your nearest emergency room.** If all of the above options are too little, too late, get emergency help.

Is It Genetic?

Bipolar disorder and cyclothymia have a significant genetic basis. They often run in families, although occasionally, they skip a generation. (If you can, find out about your grandparents' generation, too.) Bipolar I seems to have the strongest genetic basis. If you have an identical twin with bipolar disorder, the odds of having bipolar yourself are about 40 to 45 percent (Barnett and Smoller 2009). This is very high, but it also highlights the fact that genes are not the whole story. There's also a gene-and-environment interaction. Even if you have inherited a set of genes that predisposes you to bipolar, you may not develop the condition if you are not exposed to certain stressors or if you develop healthy ways of coping with stressors. Only recently have we begun to understand this gene-environment interaction, but it can be significant.

EXERCISE: FAMILY HISTORY

Has anyone in your family been diagnosed with—or do they exhibit signs or symptoms of—depression, hypomania, or mania? Use the checklist below and then write your experiences. Note that changing attitudes and knowledge about these conditions mean that information about grandparents and even aunts and uncles is likely to be limited, unless they experienced extreme symptoms. In the description column, be sure to include information about treatment and responses to treatment.

RELATIONSHIP	CLUES	DESCRIPTION
Biological Father	☑ History of depression ☑ History of mood swings, irritability, risky behavior ☑ History of alcohol or substance use ☑ History of psychiatric treatment	Father was always kind of irritable and dealt with bouts of depression. Struggled with substance abuse all his life.
Biological Mother	☐ History of depression ☑ History of mood swings, irritability, risky behavior ☐ History of alcohol or substance use ☐ History of psychiatric treatment	Mother irritable at times. Never really had an issue with alcohol or substance abuse. No psychiatric treatment. No depression as far as I know.

continued >

RELATIONSHIP	CLUES	DESCRIPTION
Biological Siblings	☐ History of depression ☐ History of mood swings, irritability, risky behavior ☐ History of alcohol or substance use ☐ History of psychiatric treatment	Only child.
Father's Parents	☑ History of depression ☑ History of mood swings, irritability, risky behavior ☑ History of alcohol or substance use ☑ History of psychiatric treatment	Dad's father was an extremely harsh alcoholic. Dad's sister believed he was manic-depressive but it wasn't talked about much back in those days.
Mother's Parents	☐ History of depression ☑ History of mood swings, irritability, risky behavior ☐ History of alcohol or substance use ☑ History of psychiatric treatment	Mom's mother had severe psychiatric issues. No alcohol or substance abuse as far as I know. Was very irritable, had extreme mood swings and engaged in risky behavior.
Other	☑ History of depression ☑ History of mood swings, irritability, risky behavior ☑ History of alcohol or substance use ☑ History of psychiatric treatment	My mother's parents' parents too: there is not much known about them. I only saw my great-grandmother once and I have no idea who my great-grandfather is. The stories passed down orally about this particular part of my family are all bad. My great-grandmother was said to have been extremely abusive and labeled by some of my grandmother's siblings as even evil.

The Bipolar Disorder–Anxiety Intersection

Bipolar disorder is a big challenge, but many people with bipolar and cyclothymia have to deal with additional challenges called "comorbidities." Of the common bipolar comorbidities, anxiety disorders and substance use disorders are the most common. We talk about substance use later in this workbook, but before we do, let's focus on the intersection between bipolar disorder and anxiety.

SOCIAL ANXIETY AND BIPOLAR DISORDER

Social anxiety is the most common anxiety disorder found in people with bipolar, which might seem strange at first, since we often associate bipolar with the outgoing and gregarious nature of hypomania and mania. But most people with bipolar have significant anxiety in social situations when they're either depressed or in a normal mood. This can be partly understood as a natural consequence of the disruption of social relationships that often occurs when someone experiences significant mood swings. If you are currently seeing a therapist, request their help with any social anxiety you are having. You can also find resources and types of therapies online (see Resources, page 154).

PTSD AND BIPOLAR DISORDER

The relationship between post-traumatic stress disorder (PTSD) and bipolar disorder is complicated but important to try to understand. Up to one-third of people with bipolar experience PTSD at some point in their lives. Psychological trauma, exposure to death or the threat of death, serious injury, or rape are among the traumatic experiences that can trigger PTSD. If you have had any of these experiences, you are at an increased risk for developing PTSD and should consult a therapist if you have access to one. Also, parents and other close family members with bipolar may inadvertently expose a child to PTSD. The alcoholic father with bipolar disorder who goes into rages, and the neglectful parents who fail to prevent their child from being exposed to abuse are just two examples of how this could play out in a family. Finally, the hypomanic and manic experiences of people with bipolar and the risk-taking behavior that often accompanies these mood states increase the risk of having traumatic events in adolescence and adulthood. Fortunately, good treatment is available that can significantly reduce PTSD symptoms. Ask your mental health professional about exposure therapy and other effective treatments.

GET ACTIVE

Throughout this book, you'll find important tips for taking care of your physical health. Building a strong and healthy body is a critical part of living well with bipolar. Believe it or not, just staying healthy can really support mood stability. For example, exercise is one of the best ways to cope with excess anxiety. Our first Whole-Health Strategy focuses on starting to build a regular exercise habit.

Exercise and Activity Planning

The best exercise is one that you can do regularly and enjoy. For mood stability, we suggest planning on 30 minutes of aerobic activity (an activity that raises your heart rate) five days a week.

Which of these activities appeals to you?

- ☒ Rapid walking or hiking
- ☐ Jogging or running
- ☐ Yoga
- ☒ A martial art (karate, jujitsu, judo, aikido, etc.)
- ☒ A racket sport (tennis, racquetball, squash, etc.)
- ☒ Swimming

- ☒ Cycling (road cycling, mountain biking, etc.)
- ☐ Circuit training
- ☐ Aerobics
- ☐ Skating
- ☐ A team sport (baseball, soccer, basketball, volleyball, etc.)
- ☐ Dancing
- ☐ A water sport (kayaking, kite skiing, open-water swimming, etc.)
- ☒ A winter sport (skiing, cross-country skiing, ice skating, etc.)
- ☐ Other: _____

Now let's figure out a schedule. Remember, 30 minutes of aerobic exercise, five days a week, is good for mood stability.

SAMPLE WEEKLY PLANNER FOR THE WEEK OF: _____

	MON	TUE	WED	THU	FRI	SAT	SUN
7:00 AM							
7:30 AM							
8:00 AM							
8:30 AM							
9:00 AM							

Notes:

PANIC AND BIPOLAR DISORDER

Almost a quarter of people with bipolar disorder also have panic disorder. If this is true for you, you know that *panic* is a sudden, overwhelming fear that makes you feel as if you were having a heart attack or even going crazy. Although a panic attack is bad enough, for many people, what's really disabling about panic attacks is the tendency to begin avoiding certain experiences in an effort to prevent having another panic attack. Unfortunately, avoidance strategies don't work in the long run; in fact, experiential avoidance is associated with an increase in panic and anxiety symptoms. The good news is that there are effective therapies that can treat panic and reverse its disabling effects. Ask your mental health professional about cognitive behavioral therapies that include graduated exposure work.

The Bipolar Disorder Effect

Bipolar disorder can have profound effects on a person's life, especially if it goes untreated. Significant mood episodes, both hypomanic and depressed, can disrupt relationships with family and friends and affect work performance.

Even more common is the shame that many people feel about their behavior, which makes it hard to reestablish contact or repair relationships after a depressive or hypomanic episode. During mood episodes, you may also miss out on opportunities for growth and development. You may have to leave school, quit a job, or go on disability. All of this may result in your feeling left behind while others in your peer group are moving on in their lives.

But it's not all bad news. As you may know from experience, bipolar II and cyclothymia can also be associated with positive skills and personality traits. Having mild hypomania sometimes leads to great productivity and creativity. In his book *The Hypomanic Edge: The Link between (a Little) Craziness and (a Lot of) Success in America*, John Gartner argues that many of this country's great accomplishments may be linked to hypomania. In a more scholarly way, Kay Redfield Jamison, in many of her works—particularly *Touched with Fire: Manic-Depressive Illness and the Artistic Temperament*—points to strong evidence of a link between bipolar and creativity.

EXERCISE: HOW HAS BIPOLAR AFFECTED YOUR LIFE?

What effects—positive and negative—has bipolar disorder or cyclothymia had on your life? Select from the list below by putting a check mark next to relevant examples, or add other examples from your personal experience.

DOMAIN	POSITIVE EFFECTS	NEGATIVE EFFECTS
Family	Receive support from family Share experiences with others who have had mood symptoms ✓ Other:_____	Loss of family relationships ✓ Strain on family relationships ✓ Misunderstanding ✓ Shame or guilt ✓ Other:_____
Friendships	Receive support from friends Share experiences with others who have had mood symptoms Other:_____	Loss of friendships ✓ Strain on friendships ✓ Misunderstanding ✓ Shame or stigma ✓ Other:_____
Intimate Relationships	Partners find the energy and creativity of hypomania appealing Receive support from partners Meet people you wouldn't ordinarily have met during hypomania Other:_____	Loss of relationships or divorce ✓ Strain on relationships ✓ Misunderstanding ✓ Shame or stigma ✓ Other:_____
Work and Financial	Energy and creativity of hypomania lead to work and financial success ✓ Creativity associated with bipolar is a key part of job or profession ✓ Other:_____	Experience discrimination or stigma ✓ Lose a job or miss out on a promotion ✓ Have to go on disability and lose income ✓ Other:_____
Health	Increased energy of hypomania leads to increased physical activity ✓ Creativity of hypomania yields more home cooking ✓ Other:_____	Substance or alcohol use problems ✓ Health problems ✓ Weight gain ✓ love to pottery Other:_____

Psychological	Feel that range of moods increases appreciation of life	Depression associated with significant pain and distress
	Struggle and success with bipolar improves psychological health	Instability of mood leads to uncertainty about self
	Other:_____	Anxiety or other symptoms that co-occur with bipolar cause impairment
		Other:_____

Takeaways and Next Steps

In this chapter, we talked about the different kinds of bipolar disorder, with an emphasis on bipolar II and cyclothymia. We reviewed the symptoms of these types of bipolar—hypomania and major depression—and talked a bit about mania, which is associated with bipolar I. Finally, we discussed the overlap of bipolar and other disorders, and the ways that bipolar disorder can affect many aspects of a person's life. Before we move on to therapeutic treatments, let's take a moment to revisit the major takeaways from this chapter.

1. Write down one or two things you learned from this chapter about the types of bipolar disorder and their symptoms.
2. Describe the symptoms of anxiety that you experience and how they relate to different mood states.
3. Identify a few action steps. For example, if you have anxiety and bipolar, what do you plan to do to get help for the anxiety symptoms you're currently experiencing?

CHAPTER TWO

Therapeutic Treatments

ALTHOUGH BIPOLAR II AND CYCLOTHYMIA ARE DIFFERENT CONDITIONS, similar therapies work for both. In this chapter, we look at the types of therapy that are effective for treating bipolar II disorder and cyclothymia, as well as the most frequently prescribed medications.

Cognitive Behavioral Therapy

Cognitive Behavioral Therapy (CBT) is a type of therapy that helps you examine how your thoughts, feelings, and behaviors are related to and interact with one another. By examining this relationship, you can explore ways to identify unhelpful thought patterns, challenge or change the way you respond to those thoughts, reinforce behaviors that support your values, help manage your symptoms, and promote overall well-being.

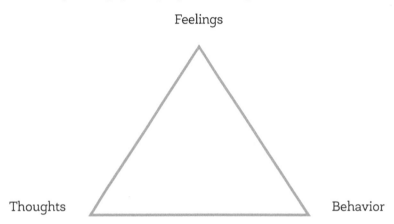

Feelings

Thoughts

Behavior

CBT techniques are useful for both depressive and energized (hypomanic) symptoms. When you are depressed, it's very common to have harmful (and often inaccurate) beliefs and thoughts that reinforce a depressed mood and interfere with taking action or engaging in activities that will improve your mood. For example, thoughts of worthlessness or guilt may lead you to isolate and withdraw from engaging in work or other social activities. Your doing so may reinforce the thought that you are worthless, causing you to definitely miss out on potentially fun or rewarding experiences—which will make you feel even worse.

A thought that can be very common with depression is "I'm a failure." CBT asks you to look at what was happening when this thought occurred. These events are called "triggers." CBT also asks you to examine the emotion you felt when you had a negative thought (feelings) and, finally, to consider how you responded to the depressive thought (behaviors).

For example, if you received negative feedback at work for turning in an assignment late, you might think, "I'm a failure," and, as a result, feel scared and sad. CBT would ask you to examine how those thoughts or feelings changed your behaviors. What did you do after having that thought? Did you avoid your boss for the rest of the day? Did you spend hours worrying instead of working? Did you generally respond in a helpful or an unhelpful way? CBT allows you to look at your thought ("I'm a failure") and your unhelpful response to that thought (avoiding work), and teaches you techniques to alter your response so that you end up with your desired outcome (completing your next assignment on time).

CBT looks at the interaction among events, thoughts, feelings, and behavior, often with a particular focus on examining and changing how we think—that's the "cognitive" part of Cognitive Behavioral Therapy. For example, CBT would ask you to examine whether the thought "I'm a failure" is helpful—is it taking you in a direction you want to go?—and also whether it is accurate. Are you really a total failure? Do other people see you that way? Or are you a person who is successful in some ways but struggles in certain areas? Does turning in an assignment late make you a complete failure? What is the evidence for and against the "failure" thought? Gradually, with practice, you replace inaccurate or self-defeating thoughts with healthier thoughts and beliefs. This process of examining and challenging your thoughts is called "cognitive restructuring."

At times, it may be difficult to identify or challenge particular thoughts, and instead, you may choose to focus on what you do in response to the thoughts (your behaviors). For example, if, when you have the thought "I'm a failure," you procrastinate the next project and avoid checking work e-mails, it may be easier for you to change the behavior than challenge the thought. You might decide to set small work goals that help you rebuild confidence, for example, working on your e-mail inbox for 10 minutes or giving yourself a half hour to set up a timeline for your next project. Better yet, offer yourself a small reward when you successfully finish creating that timeline. This kind of behavior-focused intervention can be very effective in elevating a depressed mood and is a good place to start if you're dealing with depressive thoughts that feel especially entrenched and hard to change.

When you're experiencing an episode of depression or low mood, it's also helpful to focus on behaviors that support a better mood, such as exercise, getting morning light, socializing, restricting sleep to eight hours a night, and building your sense of effectiveness by completing small, achievable tasks. Called "behavioral activation," this specific strategy is one of the most effective approaches to improving depression.

When you are in an *energized* mood state (such as hypomania), it's common to have thoughts that overestimate your abilities and underestimate the risks of your actions. These thoughts can lead to impulsive decision-making, excessive spending, and various risky behaviors.

You also can use CBT to test the accuracy of your hypomanic thinking and identify the most helpful ways to respond to it. For example, if you're thinking, "It will work out one way or another," when considering making a large purchase you can't afford, you could use CBT to gather evidence for and against the thought. Do you have the money to spend on this purchase? Are you noticing any other energized mood symptoms that would suggest this purchase is not a typical decision you would make?

Since one important feature of hypomania is reduced activity in the part of the brain that assesses risk, it can help to seek the opinions of others as well to come up with a more realistic risk assessment. Whenever you're in a hypomanic state, you may want to implement a 48-hour rule before making big decisions or purchases. Make sure to get a few good nights' sleep and consult some trusted friends or family during those 48 hours so you have more than one perspective on your decision.

EXERCISE: COGNITIVE RESTRUCTURING

Now that you're more familiar with CBT and how you can apply it to the unhelpful and possibly inaccurate thoughts that can come up when your mood is either energized or depressed, try practicing CBT's thought-analysis techniques on the thoughts in the sections below.

WHAT WAS THE SETTING FOR YOUR THOUGHTS?

When, where, and why did they happen?

_____

_____

_____

WHAT WAS YOUR MOOD?

What were you feeling when you were having these thoughts? Check the boxes for moods and rate their intensity (0–100: 0 is not intense at all, and 100 is the most intense).

☐ Numb (Intensity: _____)　　☐ Excited (Intensity: _____)

☐ Sad (Intensity: _____)　　☐ Guilty (Intensity: _____)

☐ Lonely (Intensity: _____)　　☐ Disappointed (Intensity: _____)

☐ Nervous (Intensity: _____)　　☐ Hurt (Intensity: _____)

☐ Angry (Intensity: _____)　　☐ Other: _____ (Intensity: _____)

WHAT WAS THE CONTENT OF YOUR THOUGHTS?

Write down the thoughts you were having. Try to get as close to the actual thoughts you had, rather than your summary or analysis of the thoughts; for example, "I'm a failure" rather than "I felt as though I were a failure."

_____

_____

_____

WHAT WAS THE ACCURACY OF YOUR THOUGHTS?

At the time, how sure were you that these thoughts were accurate? Write in a numeric estimate next to each thought above.

Not Sure			Completely Certain
0%		50%	100%

PROS AND CONS

What Is the Evidence for Your Thoughts?
What is the evidence for or against the thoughts? Imagine that you are summarizing arguments for a jury. What are the pros and cons?

Arguments for the thoughts:

_____

_____

_____

_____

Arguments against the thoughts:

_____

_____

_____

_____

WHAT IS A MORE BALANCED THOUGHT?

What is a more balanced thought now that you have considered the pros and cons?

_____

_____

WHAT WAS THE CONTENT OF YOUR THOUGHTS?

Now that you've taken some time to examine your thinking and consider some alternative thoughts, how has this affected your mood?

_____

_____

_____

_____

WHAT IS YOUR MOOD NOW?

Check the boxes for moods and rate their intensity (0–100: 0 is not intense at all, and 100 is the most intense).

☐ Numb (Intensity: _____)

☐ Sad (Intensity: _____)

☐ Lonely (Intensity: _____)

☐ Nervous (Intensity: _____)

☐ Angry (Intensity: _____)

☐ Excited (Intensity: _____)

☐ Guilty (Intensity: _____)

☐ Disappointed (Intensity: _____)

☐ Hurt (Intensity: _____)

☐ Other: _____ (Intensity: _____)

MEDICATIONS FOR BIPOLAR

An important treatment option for bipolar symptoms—both depression and hypomanic or energized symptoms—is certain medications called *mood stabilizers*. Choosing the right medications must involve a conversation with a clinician who has the skill and experience to provide you with effective information about the options, but the following charts may give you some useful ideas. The first chart takes a look at the types of medications and other biological treatments that may be helpful depending on your current mood state. The second chart considers which medications may be most useful on an ongoing basis to prevent episodes; it uses a rating range between one and six stars, with one star meaning less useful and six stars meaning more useful. Generally, preventing episodes is more effective than treating current symptoms.

SELECTING MEDICATIONS BY PROBLEM

TREATS HYPOMANIA AND DEPRESSION	TREATS DEPRESSION WITHOUT MOOD-DESTABILIZING EFFECTS	TREATS HYPOMANIA AND RAPID CYCLING	USE WITH CAUTION
Lithium	Lamotrigine	Atypical antipsychotics	Modafinil—for depression
Quetiapine	Fish oil	Valproate	Bright light—for depression
Olanzapine	Thyroid	Carbamazepine	Pramipexole—for depression
Carbamazepine		Lithium	TMS (transcranial magnetic stimulation)—for depression

EFFECTIVENESS IN PREVENTING EPISODES

MEDICATION	PREVENTING EPISODES	PREVENTING MANIA	PREVENTING DEPRESSION
Aripiprazole	****	****	*
Divalproex	****	**	***
Lamotrigine	****	**	***
Lithium	*****	****	**
Olanzapine	******	*****	***
Quetiapine	******	*****	***

Acceptance and Commitment Therapy

Now we turn to the next major therapy on our list of effective interventions: Acceptance and Commitment Therapy (ACT). ACT (pronounced "act") includes many techniques that can be helpful for dealing with bipolar II and cyclothymia. Psychologist Steven Hayes developed a therapeutic approach that uses acceptance and mindfulness strategies, along with a commitment to values-based behavior change, to help people foster well-being.

ACT focuses more on your *relationship* to your thoughts and emotions than on the content of your thoughts. ACT identifies core psychological processes that, when strengthened, can help reduce the distress associated with your symptoms so you can start living better. Below, we describe some of the core processes and provide techniques to help strengthen them.

ACCEPTANCE

"Acceptance," in the ACT worldview, is about accepting the reality of your current situation, whatever it may be, even when that reality is uncomfortable or distressing. That doesn't mean you give up or resign yourself to feeling unhappy. It does mean giving up the mental struggle against how things are right now because the struggle to change or reject reality is the source of much unnecessary pain and unhappiness.

Acceptance means acknowledging a situation as *it is* (instead of what our mind tells us it is or what we wish it were), even if we don't like it. This includes painful, unavoidable realities like a childhood trauma—or a bipolar diagnosis. Although it may feel self-protective, the act of struggling with or avoiding a reality that cannot be changed increases our suffering in the long run.

By allowing our experience to exist, by accepting what already is without fighting or avoiding it, we create space for the painful experience to arise and then naturally subside. We also create space to experience other, much more pleasant emotions like joy and love when we stop making our struggle with pain such a big focus of our attention.

BEING PRESENT

Present-moment awareness, also known as "mindfulness," is another ACT core process. Being present can help to manage symptoms and maintain your well-being in many ways. Dr. Jon Kabat-Zinn has defined mindfulness as "paying attention in a particular way: on purpose, in the present moment, and nonjudgmentally."

Being present increases awareness of all the thoughts, emotions, and sensations, including bipolar symptoms, that you are experiencing. In managing bipolar or cyclothymia, being present can help you identify early warning signs of mood changes and respond in a more purposeful, productive manner. If you are aware, for example, of

MINDFULNESS AS A HEALTH TOOL

Mindfulness is being used now to work with anxiety, depression, pain management, stress, and health. Research has even shown mindfulness to improve immune functioning (Davidson et al. 2003). Therefore, consider using mindfulness to promote not only your mental health, but also your physical health. Try creating a regular mindfulness practice of your own for 10 to 15 minutes a day as part of your regular self-care routine. Here are some practices to consider:

- Mindful breathing
- Mindful seeing
- Walking meditation

- Mindful appreciation
- Mindful immersion (in the present moment through day-to-day activities)

You can use the strategies included in this chapter or check out YouTube videos or apps that can help guide you through regular mindfulness practice. Your physical health—and your state of mind—will benefit!

an increase in racing thoughts, restlessness, and psychomotor agitation (purposeless motions, possibly stemming from restlessness, that can look like fidgeting, a shaking foot, or pacing), you will find it easier to notice the early signs of hypomania, which will allow you to take steps to prevent a further elevation in mood using simple strategies like prioritizing sleep and avoiding mood-altering substances.

Present-moment awareness can also help you cope with emotions such as irritability, depression, and impulsivity. It can help alleviate the suffering caused by rumination about the past and worry about the future. Being present allows you to identify what's happening in the here and now, instead of getting caught up in your thoughts, and what actions you can take *right now* to bring you closer to living the kind of life you want.

Being present means bringing awareness to the moment that you are actually living, without judging your experience as good or bad, right or wrong. It means engaging in your life with curiosity and openness for both the enjoyable moments and the more difficult ones.

Most of the exercises in this section will help you practice being mindful and present. As you work through them, note which ones you like best and might want to practice regularly as part of a plan to be present in your daily life.

EXERCISE: MINDFUL EATING

We eat many times a day, every day, and often, we consume our meals on autopilot. Mindful eating brings present awareness to this everyday activity.

To engage in mindful eating, step through each of your five senses as you prepare for and engage in eating your food: sight, sound, smell, touch, and taste. Below is a script to help guide you through one way of engaging in this practice.

- Notice what you see and describe it to yourself as you sit down with the food in front of you.
- Next, bring your attention to any sounds you experience as you move the food around. Perhaps, if there's a small object on your plate, bring your ear closer to it and notice any sounds that arise as you change its position. Remember that your thoughts may wander. If you discover this happening, acknowledge the thoughts and bring yourself back to the sensation of sound.
- Next, bring a small amount of the food up to your nose. Notice all the aromas of the food. You might also notice changes in your mouth or stomach as you experience smell.
- Next, place the first bite in your mouth without swallowing. Bring your awareness to any changes in sensations that occur when the food is inside your mouth. What does it feel like to have the food on your tongue? What textures and temperatures can you notice? Notice the taste and flavors of the food. Where do you experience these sensations in your body?
- Before you swallow, bring your awareness to what it feels like to prepare to swallow. Allow yourself to swallow, and notice any changes in sensations in your mouth, throat, and stomach. As you continue to eat, remain mindful of all the sensations that are occurring, and of course, when your mind wanders—and it will—notice that and gently return your attention to the sensations occurring as you eat in the present moment.

VALUES AND COMMITTED ACTION

Values and committed action are also among ACT's core processes. In ACT, "values" are defined as the things we cherish most and want to see more of in our lives. Values are the principles in your life that bring you a sense of meaning and significance. Values vary from person to person and can be anything from family to fitness to professional growth, depending on what you care about and want to prioritize. "Committed action" is a related idea, focused on aligning your actions with the things that are most important to you—in other words, your values. ACT guides us to choose actions that move us closer to our values as an essential part of leading a healthy, rewarding life.

WHOLE-HEALTH STRATEGY

VALUES-BASED HEALTH GOALS

Your physical health can greatly affect your mental health, and vice versa. If you are depressed, you may not be getting out of bed to exercise, and you may be eating more unhealthy foods, both of which can negatively influence your physical health. Similarly, if you are not exercising and are drinking more alcohol, this could aggravate your mood symptoms. It's also important to note that you can apply more-specific values-based health goals that target different mood states. For example, if you are depressed, engage in more aerobic activity. If you are noticing hypomanic symptoms, it might be more helpful to engage in calming exercises, such as yoga. Setting values-based goals specific to your physical health is an important part of building tools to manage your mood. Think about the various health goals you can set for this week, and get specific.

Sleep: _____

_____

(Example: This week, I will get in bed by 9:30 and discontinue all screen use.)

Physical exercise: _____

_____

(Example: I will do yoga three times a week.)

Nutrition: _____

_____

(Example: I will eat three healthy meals each day.)

Substance use: _____

_____

(Example: I will limit my alcohol to no more than one drink this week.)

Other: _____

_____

Acting in accordance with our values sounds fairly straightforward and is something most people aspire to do. But ACT recognizes that, sometimes, acting on our values can be challenging or uncomfortable. For example, if one of your values is health and you're working toward that value by exercising regularly, you may have uncomfortable experiences when you go to the gym. You might feel anxious about your current fitness level or worry that other gym-goers are judging you. These unpleasant thoughts and feelings can influence your behavior: You may start to avoid the gym and the anxious thoughts you have there. But in avoiding the gym, you are also moving away from your value of "health," which will cost you more in the long term than avoidance gains you in the short term. Committed action means acting in line with our values even when it's uncomfortable. Returning to the gym example, it means going there to work out, despite feeling anxious.

EXERCISE: IDENTIFYING YOUR VALUES
AND COMMITTED ACTIONS

This exercise will help you identify the values that are most important to you and then create committed-action goals in line with your values.

Begin by placing a number 1, 2, or 3 next to each value: 1 means the value is not important to you, 2 signifies an important value, and 3 points to a very important value. Focus on what matters most to you—not what you think your friends, family, or colleagues might choose, but what you yourself value most.

___ Community	___ Love	___ Balance	___ Justice
___ Friendship	___ Respect	___ Determination	___ Pleasure
___ Leadership	___ Authenticity	___ Honesty	___ Spirituality
___ Religion	___ Authority	___ Optimism	___ Challenge
___ Achievement	___ Creativity	___ Self-Respect	___ Fame
___ Compassion	___ Happiness	___ Beauty	___ Kindness
___ Competency	___ Loyalty	___ Fairness	___ Popularity
___ Fun	___ Responsibility	___ Humor	___ Stability
___ Learning	___ Autonomy	___ Peace	___ Family
___ Reputation	___ Curiosity	___ Service	___ Knowledge
___ Adventure	___ Health	___ Boldness	___ Purpose
___ Contribution	___ Openness	___ Faith	___ Wealth
___ Growth	___ Security		

After identifying which values are most important to you (the ones you rated a 3), choose the 10 values you most want to work on. If you have fewer than 10 values with a 3 rating, pick all of them. Now, in the table below, rate how closely your current actions align with each value on a scale from 1 to 10, with 1 meaning your actions aren't at all consistent with the value, and 10 meaning your actions are fully in line with the value.

Next, of the values you've discovered your current behavior is not supporting, pick your top three targets for change. What actions can you take this week that will bring you closer to those values? For example, if one of your values is "friendship," you might decide to reach out to two friends this week and make plans. By the time you've finished the steps in this values exercise, you will have created a customized action plan for change.

	VALUE	HOW MUCH YOU'RE LIVING THE VALUE (1 TO 10)	ACTIONS TO TAKE THIS WEEK THAT BRING YOU CLOSER TO THAT VALUE
1			
2			
3			
4			
5			
6			
7			
8			
9			
10			

COGNITIVE DEFUSION

In our discussion of CBT, we talked about recognizing unhelpful thoughts and replacing them with more helpful ones, using a technique called cognitive restructuring. ACT helps us deal with unhelpful thoughts in a different way, through a process called "cognitive defusion."

One of the things that makes problematic thoughts difficult to change, "fix," or even notice is that our thoughts present themselves as reflections of reality. In other words, our thoughts present themselves as facts. ACT teaches us that thoughts are *not* facts; they are our mental interpretations of events. Thoughts are colored by our motivations, our emotional state, and our personal history.

Our thoughts, especially the inaccurate or unhelpful ones, can cause us problems when we respond to them as if they *were* facts. Consider the example of a young child whose parents told him he was chubby. As a result, he grew up frequently thinking, "I'm fat." By the time he reached adulthood, he had fully identified with thoughts of being fat. As an adult, he thinks of himself as a fat person rather than as a person who has the thought, "I'm fat." This identification with the "I'm fat" thought could even persist after he has crash-dieted to an unhealthy level of thinness. In ACT, this overidentification with thoughts is called "cognitive fusion."

Cognitive defusion helps you see your thoughts more objectively, recognizing them as creations of the mind that come and go, rather than as fixed external realities. As we become less fused with our thoughts, we can break the pattern of reacting automatically to them without pausing to consider whether they are accurate or helpful.

Defusion helps us shift our relationship with our thinking, "unhooking" us from particularly painful, inaccurate, or unhelpful thoughts. It allows us to take a step back and observe the thoughts from a bit of a distance, almost as though they were floating by like leaves on a stream.

One simple defusion technique involves naming a problematic thought for what it is: a thought. Let's consider the example of a thought common to people experiencing a depressive episode: "I can't get out of bed." To reduce the power of the thought on your behavior, you can reframe the thought this way: "I am having the thought that I can't get out of bed" or even "I am noticing I'm having the thought that I can't get out of bed." Over time, this cognitive defusion practice will make it easier to put your feet on the floor despite the thought that you can't. Try the exercise below to practice cognitive defusion.

EXERCISE: THOUGHT DEFUSION

Start by picking a thought that may be a bit "sticky"—a thought that can get in the way of doing something helpful for your physical or mental health—and write it below.

Sticky Thought
(Example: No one will like me.)

_____

_____

_____

_____

Now try writing (and saying out loud), "I'm having the thought that . . ."
(Example: I'm having the thought that no one will like me.)

_____

_____

_____

_____

Now try writing (and saying out loud), "I notice I'm having the thought that . . ."
(Example: I notice I'm having the thought that no one will like me.)

_____

_____

_____

_____

Now try defusing that thought even further by noticing yourself notice you are having the thought. (Example: I notice that I'm noticing that I'm having the thought that no one will like me.)

_____

_____

_____

_____

How has this process changed your relationship to the thought? Does it seem less powerful? Less "real"? Do you think it would be easier to resist the sticky thought?

_____

_____

_____

_____

CBT and ACT's cognitive defusion practices can help you reduce your overall stress. As you have been learning, how you interpret your thoughts affects how you experience them. For example, if you have the thought, "I will never get through this work assignment" or "I can't do this," and you believe this thought is a fact, you'll experience more stress when you work on the assignment. If you use defusion and cognitive restructuring techniques, you'll experience less stress and feel more confident. The more you practice these techniques, the better equipped you will feel to manage the stress and symptoms of bipolar and cyclothymia.

Takeaways and Next Steps

In this chapter, we have explored three types of therapies that can help you live well with bipolar. We considered the relationship among thoughts, emotions, and behavior and explored some techniques from Cognitive Behavioral Therapy (CBT) that you can use to deal with depression and hypomania. We briefly considered some of the medications that may be useful as part of your intervention plan. And we spent a fair amount of time exploring some of the ideas from ACT (acceptance, values and committed action, and cognitive defusion). If these tools seem useful, you will want to practice them and read more about them. See the Resources section (page 154) for more information.

RATE THESE TOOLS

TOOL	USEFULNESS NOW (0 TO 5)	DESIRE TO READ MORE (0 TO 5)	POSSIBLE READING SOURCES
Cognitive Restructuring			
Medications			
Acceptance			
Committed Action			
Cognitive Defusion			

CHAPTER THREE

Finding Your Baseline: How Are You Right Now?

DEVELOPING A PLAN FOR DEALING WITH BIPOLAR effectively begins with an assessment of how you are functioning in all the important areas of your life. We are strong believers in the idea that successful change generally begins with a clear idea of where you are at the beginning of the process. That said, self-assessment is often surprisingly difficult.

You may think you know all about your moods, or you may be sick and tired of thinking about the impact of bipolar on your life. We know how you feel. And yet we also know that a thoughtful self-assessment is essential as you build a new life for yourself. A favorite author and wise psychologist, Carl Rogers, taught us many years ago that if you are to change, you must know, and accept, your starting point and that once you do accept where you are now, change begins to happen naturally. In chapter 2, we talked about acceptance, an important concept that will play a role in many aspects of your recovery.

Overall Functioning

The World Health Organization has developed a set of questions to assess functioning across important life domains and to measure the effect of health conditions on functioning. We will use those questions as a framework for reviewing how you're doing now.

COGNITIVE FUNCTIONING

Even experienced psychiatrists may be unaware of the profound impact that bipolar and cyclothymia can have on cognitive functioning. Only recently, one of us was reviewing records from a colleague and noticed that he had felt compelled to notify the Department of Motor Vehicles that due to her impairment on a standard cognitive test of memory, his bipolar patient also had dementia. However, two months later, the patient was no longer depressed, and her cognitive functioning returned to normal. This lack of professional awareness of the full range of bipolar symptoms, while not unusual, had a profound effect on his patient, who lost her license and had to spend months convincing the DMV that she really could drive when she wasn't clinically depressed. In our clinic, we have begun to routinely perform neurocognitive testing so we can show our patients how their cognitive functioning is related to mood.

On tests of cognitive functioning, people with depression tend to say they can't remember the answers to test questions and they lose the ability to multitask and stay focused. They give lots of "I don't know" answers on such tests. They may even fear they are experiencing dementia symptoms.

It's not just depression that affects cognitive functioning. Hypomania also has its impact, but these effects are harder to see. Unlike someone with depression, who will answer, "I don't know" or "I don't remember," the hypomanic person will answer questions even if they don't know the answer, and they won't know they are guessing.

EXERCISE: COGNITIVE SELF-ASSESSMENT

Here are some questions to ask yourself about your current cognitive functioning. Read each question and then assign a number from 1 to 5 for each, depending on how much you feel your symptoms are affecting you in that area. Rating key: 1 is severely impaired, 3 is somewhat impaired, and 5 is not impaired.

____ How much difficulty do you have staying focused on a task for 10 minutes? For example, can you read a chapter in a book without distraction?

____ Do you have trouble remembering to do important things? People with depression often get so worried about their memory that their anxiety actually makes them forgetful. On the other hand, people with hypomania forget important things without being as concerned about their forgetfulness as they should be.

____ How much difficulty do you have analyzing problems and finding solutions? If you're feeling depressed, you're likely to get bogged down in the details. Hypomania leads to coming up with answers that don't consider all the important factors.

____ Is it hard for you to learn new skills? This tends to be a problem for many people who are depressed or anxious.

____ Do you have trouble understanding what other people are saying? Again, depression can get in the way of understanding, because you may be too worried to really focus on what the other person is saying. If you're hypomanic, you'll tend to have trouble staying focused on what the other person is saying for long enough to understand, and you may assume you know what they're going to say, without really listening to the details.

____ Finally, how much trouble do you have communicating with others? If you're depressed, you will find it hard to come up with anything to say, and you may give single-word answers to complex questions. If you're hypomanic, you may have trouble slowing your thoughts down so you can communicate effectively. You may jump from idea to idea and have trouble translating those thoughts into sentences.

Add up your total.

A SCORE OF . . .	MEANS YOU FEEL YOU ARE . . .
6 to 12	Severely cognitively impaired
13 to 18	Moderately cognitively impaired
19 to 24	Mildly cognitively impaired
25 to 30	Minimally cognitively impaired

WORK LIFE

It's easy to see how these cognitive difficulties could make it hard to function in a job. Many people with bipolar are creative and intelligent but have trouble performing consistently in the work environment. They may find it difficult to handle the day-to-day stresses of a job; alternatively, they may be able to do remarkable work at one point in a mood cycle but be completely unable to finish tasks at another point. For this reason, people with bipolar may need to find ways of working in environments where they don't always have to be consistent—for example, doing contract work where they can set their own schedule or finding an employer who understands that, as with many chronic medical conditions, there may be times when the employee is not as successful or effective. If you have found that not working, or working limited hours, is best for you, that's perfectly fine. The following questions are for those who spend some part of their week in a workplace setting, although if you are not working, you could do this exercise by considering your learning goals (school success) and other personal development goals (volunteer work).

Using the same scale as before—in which 1 is severely impaired, 3 is somewhat impaired, and 5 is not impaired—rate your overall level of functioning in your work life. This exercise is not about how you are doing based on external standards for success; it's about how you are doing based on your own personal values and goals.

____ How much difficulty have you had achieving your educational goals? Have you had to leave an educational program or school before gaining a degree? Have you had to abandon a training program?

____ How much trouble have you had achieving your professional goals? Have you had to leave a job because of bipolar? Have you changed to a lower-paying job or one that's less satisfying because of difficulty managing stress? Have you had trouble finding a volunteer position that is satisfying and meets your personal goals and needs?

____ How much difficulty have you experienced in your work or professional relationships? Have you found it hard to establish and maintain good relationships with coworkers, with a boss, with customers?

Add up your total.

A SCORE OF . . .	MEANS YOU FEEL YOU ARE . . .
3 to 5	Severely impaired
6 to 9	Moderately impaired
10 to 12	Mildly impaired
13 or above	Minimally impaired

SELF-CARE

How are you doing at taking care of yourself? Daily habits are very important for people with bipolar. Regular sleep routines play a key role in mood stability but are often a challenge to maintain. Diet and exercise also can play a key role in enhancing mood stability. Self-care also means taking care of your overall health by actively addressing any health issues you have, rather than putting off needed care.

Here are some questions to ask yourself about your current level of self-care. Read each question and then assign a number from 1 to 5 for each, depending on how much you feel your symptoms are affecting you in that area. Rating key: 1 is severely impaired, 3 is somewhat impaired, and 5 is not impaired.

___ How much difficulty do you have taking care of basic needs on your own? Do you have trouble keeping up with showering and washing? For many people who are depressed, these "simple" tasks become overwhelming and feel impossible.

___ How much trouble do you have doing basic housework, cleaning your clothes, shopping, and preparing food? Again, depression tends to have a bigger impact on these aspects of functioning. Keeping your home neat, even making your bed regularly, can be a big mood boost and also reduce your anxiety.

___ Are you keeping regular sleep hours that fit your work schedule and meet your needs for sleep? People with bipolar often stay up too late. This pattern can feel natural and normal but may contribute to poorer mood health.

___ How is your diet? A healthy diet leads to a strong body and greater reserves of natural energy, but many people with bipolar find themselves drawn to a diet of too much sugar and simple carbohydrates like white flour. If you aren't vegetarian, eating fish at least twice a week and plenty of fresh fruit and vegetables can improve mood stability.

___ People with bipolar tend to have more physical health problems, but they also may have trouble making doctor's appointments. How well are you dealing with your need for health care? Do you have a primary care doctor? Have you been putting off visits to see a doctor?

Add up your total.

A SCORE OF . . .	MEANS YOU FEEL YOU ARE . . .
5 to 10	Severely impaired
11 to 15	Moderately impaired
16 to 20	Mildly impaired
21 to 25	Minimally impaired

INTIMATE RELATIONSHIPS

Intimate relationships are frequently strained by mood ups and downs. Our partners can often see things we may not notice. Their observations can serve as an early warning system for mood instability. In our clinic, it's rare for someone who is hypomanic to seek treatment unless they are encouraged to do so by a partner. While most people with bipolar or cyclothymia find depression to be more disturbing than hypomania, intimate partners are often challenged more by hypomania. The impulsive decision-making, self-preoccupation, and risk-taking of hypomania are exhausting, as well as the hyperactive energy.

How much difficulty do you have getting along with people who are close to you? How much of a strain have your relationships been under due to bipolar or cyclothymia? Have any relationships ended, at least in part, due to your mood swings and other symptoms?

Using the same scale as before—in which 1 is severely impaired, 3 is somewhat impaired, and 5 is not impaired—rate your overall level of functioning in your intimate relationships.

_____ How much difficulty do the consequences of your ups and downs create in your intimate relationships? Have partners been unsupportive? Have mood symptoms prompted arguments?

_____ How much trouble have you had sustaining intimate relationships? Have relationships ended because of bipolar?

_____ How much trouble have you had developing intimate relationships? Have you found it difficult to get to know new people? Have you ended up in relationships with people who were not a good choice?

_____ Are you able to get support from your intimate relationships when you're in need? Have you been able to talk to partners about your private fears, mood symptoms, and so on?

_____ Overall, how satisfied are you with the quality of your relationships over time?

Add up your total.

A SCORE OF...	MEANS YOU FEEL YOU ARE...
5 to 9	Severely impaired
10 to 15	Moderately impaired
16 to 20	Mildly impaired
21 to 25	Minimally impaired

FAMILY RELATIONSHIPS

Family relationships are also frequently disrupted. Family members are often unable to understand the diagnosis of bipolar II or cyclothymia. They may express the concern that the diagnosis can't be accurate because they have never seen any manic behavior. They may not understand the impairment that can result from milder mood swings.

Take a moment to reflect: Are there strains in your family relationships? Do any of your family members have misconceptions about your diagnosis?

Rate your overall level of functioning in your family relationships: 1 is severely impaired, 3 is somewhat impaired, and 5 is not impaired.

____ How much difficulty do the effects of your ups and downs create in your family relationships? Have family members been unsupportive? Have you ended up having arguments because of mood symptoms?

____ Have you had trouble sustaining family relationships? Have relationships ended or become distant due to the effects of bipolar?

____ Are you able to get support from your family when you're in need? Do you have someone you can talk to about your private fears, mood symptoms, and so on?

____ Overall, how satisfied are you with the quality of your family relationships over time?

Add up your total.

A SCORE OF . . .	MEANS YOU FEEL YOU ARE . . .
4 to 7	Severely impaired
8 to 12	Moderately impaired
13 to 16	Mildly impaired
17 or above	Minimally impaired

MOOD CHARTING

For many of us, it's difficult to have a clear picture of how our moods change over time. It's only by tracking our moods that we can see what influences them and how we can achieve greater mood stability. Being comfortable thinking about your moods daily, in a reflective and nonjudgmental way, is a foundation for healthy living.

"Mood charting" is a way to keep track of your mood fluctuations over time. There are many online solutions you can use. However, if you choose to keep a mood chart, we recommend that your chart consider these factors:

- Keep it as simple as possible. The essentials involve tracking sleep, mood, and important events. Mood charting should take just a couple of minutes a day if you want it to become a long-term habit.

- Balance the need to share your chart and the need to keep it confidential. Ideally, a mood chart should be shared with your therapist or psychiatrist, but

you should have confidence that the information won't go any further. Think carefully about free smartphone apps and whether you can trust the security of the information.

- Set up a daily alarm and keep a commitment to fill in your mood chart when the alarm goes off. Or, if your life is too complicated to allow you to do it at the same time every day, set up two reminders and commit to doing it when the second alarm goes off, if you were unable to do it at the first alarm.

- Reward yourself for your consistency.

Here are some examples of apps and other tools you can use to incorporate mood charting into your routine. https://moodsurfing.com/links-and-apps/

SOCIAL LIFE

Friendships and a strong support network are important foundations of everyone's mental health, but these relationships can also be affected by bipolar. Depression can seem like a burden to friends if a relationship becomes more about taking care of the person with bipolar or cyclothymia than a relationship of equal participants. The periodic disappearance of the friend with bipolar (when they become depressed, for example) may lead to strain in the relationship, or even the ending of the relationship. Either way, maintaining a support network and healthy friendships is likely to require extra effort from you.

Consider how well you are doing at maintaining a good social network. Do you have someone you can talk to about difficult topics such as depression and feelings of hopelessness? Do you work to strengthen your friendships and make sure there's a healthy give-and-take in them? Is this an area where you'd like to see improvement in your life?

Rate your overall level of functioning in your social life: 1 is severely impaired, 3 is somewhat impaired, and 5 is not impaired.

___ How much difficulty do the effects of your ups and down create in your friendships and other social relationships? Have friends been unsupportive? Have you had arguments because of mood symptoms?

___ Have you had trouble sustaining friendships and other social relationships? Have relationships ended or become distant due to the effects of bipolar?

___ Can you get support from your social relationships when you're in need? Do you have someone you can talk to about your fears, mood symptoms, and so on?

___ Overall, how satisfied are you with the quality of your friendships and other social relationships over time?

Add up your total.

A SCORE OF . . .	MEANS YOU FEEL YOU ARE . . .
4 to 7	Severely impaired
8 to 12	Moderately impaired
13 to 16	Mildly impaired
17 or above	Minimally impaired

Stages of Recovery

A useful framework for thinking about where you are in the process of recovery draws on something called the Stages of Change Model, developed by James Prochaska and Carlo DiClemente in 1983. This has become the way many mental health professionals think about recovery from substance use disorders, but it's useful for all sorts of challenges, including bipolar II and cyclothymia. The model divides the process of coming to terms with a problem into stages; this helps you think about what you should do to move forward at each step in the process.

We have modified the Stages of Change Model slightly to make it more relevant to the unique challenges of dealing with bipolar II and cyclothymia.

STAGE 1: PRE-CONTEMPLATION

In the pre-contemplation stage, you wouldn't be thinking about bipolar disorder—so this probably isn't you. You wouldn't be reading this workbook, because it wouldn't seem relevant to you. People around you might have expressed concern about your mood swings, but you would be pretty sure that your ups and downs didn't have anything to do with bipolar. You might be resistant to the idea of bipolar disorder because of some misunderstanding of what it means, perhaps a fear that it would mean you're "crazy." You might feel resigned to your mood swings and, out of a sense of hopelessness, deliberately avoid thinking about them. Or you might rationalize the ups and downs as responses to events, nothing more than what anyone would experience if they faced the same challenges.

Whatever your situation, the next step would be to increase your awareness and begin to consider your mood instability a problem that may have a solution. The challenge for those around you would be to understand that the pre-contemplation stage is a normal part of the process of coming to grips with any new and serious problem.

STAGE 2: CONTEMPLATION

You enter the contemplation stage when you first begin to consider the possibility that you might have bipolar disorder or cyclothymia. Most people in this stage are on the fence about what to do. They're not ready to change, and they feel the need to gather more information about the condition and its treatment. You might be at that point right now if you are reading this workbook, but you're still not really convinced that it applies to you or you aren't sure that thinking of your mood swings in this way will be beneficial. The main task at this stage is to gather information.

People in the contemplation stage go from thinking about the losses associated with change ("If I say I'm bipolar, it means I'll have to take medication for the rest of my life" or "If I am bipolar, people will think I'm crazy") to thinking about the gains. When you start to think there might be a better life ahead of you if you get help coping with mood swings ("Maybe if I get help for bipolar, my relationship will be better" or "Perhaps I don't have to suffer from these depressive periods any longer"), then you're getting ready for the planning stage.

STAGE 3: PLANNING

The planning stage would be a good time to begin reading this workbook. In the planning stage, you are committed to making a change, you have accepted that you have a problem with mood swings, and you are figuring out what you will need to do to deal with the problem. This is an important stage. If you are going to deal effectively with the challenges of bipolar, you want to devote some time to thinking through your plan. This workbook will help you do that.

STAGE 4: ACTIVE PHASE—CRISIS RESOLUTION

Once you have a plan, you move into the stage of taking action. You might contact a therapist or psychiatrist. For many people, this happens because of a crisis. Perhaps a very severe depression has caused the crisis, or maybe a partner or family member insists you get help. If this is true for you, the first thing you must do is address the crisis. If you are depressed and perhaps suicidal, you need to get help so you don't feel so overwhelmed and alone.

In a crisis, you can't think clearly about the long-term plan. You should focus on finding the right kind of support. Seek a therapist with expertise in treating bipolar, or find a good psychiatrist.

HEALTHY DIET PLANNER

A healthy diet is an important part of living well with bipolar II or cyclothymia. You want to make sure you are getting all the nutrients that will support a healthy brain. Many people with depression find themselves craving high-carbohydrate foods (sweets, sugars, white bread, pasta, and so on). Unfortunately, indulging this craving can create a vicious cycle that may lead to gradual weight gain and chronic low-level inflammation.

The diet that has been the best studied and shown to be helpful for people with bipolar is the Mediterranean diet (see, for example, Parletta et al. 2017).

The Mediterranean diet is based on the traditional diet of rural people living in Greece, Italy, and the Mediterranean islands. It's rich in olive oil, fresh fruits, vegetables, nuts, fish, and legumes (beans). It does not include sodas, spreadable fats (such as margarine, butter, and mayonnaise), red meat, and commercial sweets (sweet baked goods and candies).

You can use this worksheet to track how closely you are following the diet. (You might want to make copies of this sheet to track your diet over additional weeks.) Daily, you should get four tablespoons of olive oil, three servings of fresh fruits, and two servings of vegetables. Weekly, try for three servings of nuts, three servings of fish, three servings of legumes, and two servings of a tomato sauce called Sofrito (feel free to substitute other tomato sauces).

HEALTHY DIET PLANNER

	MON	TUE	WED	THUR	FRI	SAT	SUN
Olive Oil: 4 tablespoons							
Fresh Fruits: 3 servings/day							
Vegetables: 2 servings/day							
Nuts: 3 servings/week							
Fish: 3 servings/week							
Legumes: 3 servings/week							
Sofrito: 2 servings/week							
Sodas < 1/day							
Spreadable Fats < 1 serving/day							
Red and Processed Meat < 1 serving/day							
Commercial Sweets < 3 servings/week							

(Diet planner courtesy of moodsurfing.com)

STAGE 5: ACTIVE PHASE—BUILDING A FOUNDATION

Most people who have bipolar or cyclothymia have suffered losses because of their mood swings. They may have had to pass up professional opportunities or may have lost relationships or friendships. It's easy to focus on those losses and to want to find a way of recovering them. But it's important to start by building a foundation of mood stability. Let's consider an example:

John is a very bright young man who has been working in computer start-ups as a software engineer. Year after year, he finds a new job and throws himself into making a success of it. The pay is good, and the potential rewards of stock options offer the hope that he can make up for several years of jobs that didn't work out. Unfortunately, in each case, he slips into depression and the excessive drinking that goes with it—and soon he must find another job.

The lure of the "quick fix" is a constant challenge for people with bipolar. For John, building a foundation for recovery meant accepting the fact that alcohol was a problem, not a solution, and committing to sobriety. It also meant recognizing that staying up all night playing video games and then trying to go to work the next day was not something his body could tolerate. He needed to develop a more regular sleep cycle and find a balance between distraction and work. He didn't have to give up excitement and creativity, but he had to find a sustainable balance.

It took a year to make these changes and a fair amount of support from a good therapist, but out of this process, he built a solid foundation that allowed him to succeed at work. And with that foundation in place, his natural ability helped him make up much of the lost time of early adulthood.

This workbook is about building a strong foundation of healthy habits that can lead to increased mood stability and pave the way to success.

STAGE 6: ACTIVE PHASE—LIVING WELL

In the midst of the turbulence your mood disorder can cause, sometimes it's hard to see that there is hope for more than just a short period of stability followed by another crisis. It has been our privilege to help many people move from building a foundation to living well. "Living well" does not mean experiencing no ups and downs. It does mean, however, that the ups and downs don't threaten relationships, career, or other life goals that are important to you.

For many people, it means being able to take advantage of the promise of their creativity and passion. This is the reward for doing the work that we outline in this workbook.

LAPSES AND RELAPSES

Wherever you are in the process of recovery, it's always wise to recognize the possibility of a recurrence. Having a strong plan in place and being clear about the warning signs will allow you to weather the storm, but some amount of awareness or vigilance about mood swings is usually the price of long-term success. Later in this workbook, we talk about how to develop a crisis plan (page 96). The goal of this plan is to make sure that any recurrence is brief and doesn't upset the foundation you have built. (Note that a recurrence is known as a "lapse," rather than a "relapse," in the terminology of the Stages of Change Model.)

EXERCISE: FIND YOUR BASELINE

What are you like when you are well? For some people with bipolar, this question seems unanswerable: They have been dealing with mood swings throughout their life. But many people have experienced periods of stability, and it can be helpful to remember what you were like during those times. Your focus as you think about this question should be on a period of stability rather than a time of unusual brilliance and success, which might really be hypomania. Focus on a time when you could sustain good friendships and relationships, and try to create a picture in your mind of what that time was like. Now describe that time. "When I am well, I . . ."

_____

_____

_____

_____

_____

_____

Five-Year Plan

Now that you have thought about where to begin the process of recovery, and before we move on to discussing the how-tos of living well with bipolar or cyclothymia, it makes sense to think about your vision for the future. Where are you now? And five years from now, if you implement the plan that you create with the help of this workbook, what do you want your life to look like? After you have filled in these two columns, fill in intermediate goals for one month (in order to kick off the process with an early success, make this goal an easy one to accomplish), one year, and two years.

	NOW	1 MONTH	1 YEAR	2 YEARS	5 YEARS
Physical Health					
Mental Health					
Spiritual					
Social					
Family					
Romantic					
Professional					
Financial					
Housing					

Takeaways and Next Steps

In this chapter, we looked at the important, and potentially challenging, assessment of where you are now. If you completed the exercises, give yourself a big "Congratulations!"—this is hard work.

We also reviewed how you can apply the Stages of Change Model to recovery from bipolar. At every stage in the process, there are important tasks to work on, whether it's learning more about bipolar, developing a plan for change, or beginning to implement that change.

We talked about the importance of mood charting, a concept you will hear about several times in this workbook.

Before we dive into the details of coping with bipolar II and cyclothymia, let's take a moment to identify the most important things you learned in this chapter.

What are the key areas of functioning that you want to see improve? Rate them from 0 (least important to you) to 5 (most important to you).

___ Cognitive functioning

___ Work and school functioning

___ Self-care

___ Intimate relationships

___ Family relationships

___ Social support and friendships

What steps will you take in the next month to begin to implement your five-year plan?

_____

_____

_____

_____

_____

_____

PART TWO

Managing Hypomania & Depression

In this part of the workbook, we talk about strategies for managing some of the symptoms that commonly occur during energized states such as hypomania. While hypomania may be a welcome respite from depression, it creates its own set of risks and is often the mood state that partners find the hardest to cope with. Using the tools in this part for managing energized states will minimize the negative effects. Remember to make some copies of the exercises before filling them in so you can use them again later.

CHAPTER FOUR

The Experience of Hypomania

ONE OF THE MOST CHALLENGING THINGS ABOUT HYPOMANIA is that people often enjoy the experience—at least at first. The early symptoms, including euphoria, grandiosity, and racing thoughts, can be a pleasurable rush. But as you may already know, there are downsides such as irritability, agitation, and impulsivity. If you recognize that you are moving into an energized mood, focus on behavioral interventions that support you in stabilizing your mood and that reduce the risks of impulsive or risky behaviors.

In this chapter, you will read about several strategies that may be useful for particular situations. Overall, though, you will want to focus on a few strategies that are particularly important and effective in managing hypomania:

- Prioritize sleep—aim for eight consecutive hours.
- Avoid caffeine and other substances that can further destabilize your mood.
- Engage in calming activities such as meditation, warm baths, listening to calming music, and so on.
- Create a 48-hour rule, where you wait before making important decisions.
- Avoid activities that may promote further excitement or conflict.
- Consider contacting your therapist or medication providers.
- Consider buying and using blue-blocking glasses.

BLUE-BLOCKING GLASSES

Research has shown that blue light indicates daytime to the brain. It is the portion of the light spectrum that affects circadian rhythms (the internal clock) most strongly. While the eye captures blue light through sunlight, it can also be received through electronic devices. Nighttime lights, including TV monitors, smartphones, and computer screens, are full of blue light. Blue-blocking glasses block blue light from the eye, so by wearing them in the evening, you might be able to reduce energized mood symptoms by blocking out this part of the spectrum and reducing the impact of artificial light from devices (Zagorski 2016).

Grandiosity and Euphoria

When you experience an energized mood, it's common to feel an unusual sense of confidence and well-being—we call those feelings "grandiosity" and "euphoria." When you're experiencing them, you may find that you minimize the risks of your choices, and you may make decisions that focus on immediate pleasure, without considering the consequences.

It's important to recognize this mood shift early, in order to prevent negative consequences. For example, while feeling too confident about your ability to complete tasks in a short period of time, you may take on too many projects, only to find that you fail to complete them, resulting in negative effects on your relationships or career. Or you may decide to start a new business, invest money, or make big purchases in a way that turns out to be unwise.

After experiencing depression, you may find the sense of well-being and increased confidence accompanying many energized mood states to be a welcome relief. The reduction of self-critical and negative thoughts can, in fact, free you up to do more, but it's hard to avoid the potential negative consequences of overly optimistic choices. Also, for many people, the longer and more intense your hypomanic state, the deeper the depression that follows it.

RECOGNIZING WARNING SIGNS

EXERCISE: IDENTIFYING SIGNS OF GRANDIOSITY AND EUPHORIA

Below is a chart to help you identify past thoughts and behaviors associated with experiencing grandiosity and euphoria. Try filling this out when you are not in an energized state. Also, consider asking others for input related to past behaviors they have seen in you.

	EXAMPLES OF PAST THOUGHTS	EXAMPLES OF PAST BEHAVIORS
Self-Confidence	I can do this better than anyone else.	I tried to remodel my kitchen alone and ruined the flooring.
Interest in Having Fun	I'll never have this opportunity again.	I stayed out all night without sleeping, and my mood got worse.
Sense of Humor	They think I'm hysterical.	I made inappropriate jokes at work and got a written warning.

continued >

	EXAMPLES OF PAST THOUGHTS	EXAMPLES OF PAST BEHAVIORS
Overoptimistic Outlook on the Future	It will all work out, no matter what.	I quit my job without having another one lined up or any savings.
Reduced Concern for Consequences	I don't care what he thinks.	I took my roommate's car without asking.
Other Examples, e.g., "taking physical risks"		

THE BIPOLAR DISORDER WORKBOOK

EXERCISE: RESTRUCTURING THOUGHTS

Of the thoughts you identified above, which ones led to behaviors that had negative consequences? As we practiced in chapter 2, try using CBT to evaluate and restructure the following thoughts.

SITUATION (the event leading up to the feeling)	I walked into my kitchen and wanted to redecorate it.			
EMOTION OR FEELING (name the emotions and their strength from 0% to 100 %)	Excitement 90%			
AUTOMATIC THOUGHT	I can do this better than anyone else.			
EVIDENCE THAT SUPPORTS THE THOUGHT	I am a creative person. I have learned how to fix things on YouTube in the past.			
EVIDENCE THAT DOES NOT SUPPORT THE THOUGHT	I have never changed plumbing and flooring in the past. I have taken on home improvements before, when energized, that haven't turned out well.			
ALTERNATIVE THOUGHT	I'm going to wait and research this further to see if I can get support from someone with experience before taking action.			
EMOTION OR FEELING	Excitement 45%			

NEW APPROACHES TO THOUGHTS AND BEHAVIORS

Now that you are aware of thoughts and behaviors that occurred in the past when you experienced grandiosity and euphoria, you can use this awareness to respond differently when these feelings arise again. You began working toward this in the last exercise, by practicing restructuring your thoughts.

You may find it helpful to use the ACT tools we discussed in chapter 2, such as mindfulness, defusion, and values-based committed action.

Defusion and mindfulness are helpful when you first notice the warning signs of grandiosity and euphoria, for example, noticing that you are thinking, "I can do anything," and realizing that this is a thought, not a fact. Using the strategies of cognitive defusion, you can let the thought pass without acting on it and without potentially saying or doing things you'll regret.

EXERCISE: USING COGNITIVE DEFUSION TO MANAGE HYPOMANIA

Try practicing the technique you learned earlier: naming a thought as a thought. Begin by identifying an unhelpful thought you had in the past when your mood was energized.

_____

Now try writing (and saying out loud), "I'm having the thought that . . ."

_____

Now try writing (and saying out loud), "I notice that I'm having the thought that . . ."

_____

_____

Now try defusing that thought even further by noticing yourself notice you are having the thought. "I notice that I'm noticing that I'm having the thought that . . ."

_____

_____

_____

The other defusion strategy is naming the thought. For example, the thought "I can do anything" can be defused by naming it: "That is grandiosity" or "Grandiosity is here." The same can be done with irritability, frustration, and anxiety; for example, "Worry—there is worry." Of the thoughts you identified earlier, try naming one below.

The thought:

_____

_____

How you would name the thought:

_____

Some of the past behaviors you listed in the Restructuring Thoughts exercise (page 61) have probably caused you to act in ways that are not aligned with your values. Take a moment to consider this and how you might minimize the extent to which your mood cycles can get you offtrack.

If you instead focused on values-based action when you are energized or hypomanic, how would that be different from past choices? For example, if you identified health and family as top values in the Identifying Your Values and Committed Actions exercise (page 30), which committed actions (health-focused behaviors) could you engage in to reinforce mood stability?

Look at the list of strategies for dealing with an energized mood at the beginning of this chapter (page 57) and think about which ones might be useful in the future. After reviewing the list, fill out the coping plan below.

"If I notice the following grandiose or euphoric thoughts or behaviors are occurring . . ."

_____

_____

_____

_____

"I plan to implement the following coping strategies . . ."

_____

_____

_____

_____

Racing Thoughts

"Racing thoughts" is a shorthand term to describe an increase in the speed, number, and diversity of the kinds of thoughts that occur during energized periods like hypomania. As your thoughts become faster, it can be difficult to keep up with them. You may find that you are talking faster, and other people may have a hard time understanding you, especially if you start jumping from one idea to the next. Racing thoughts can also interfere with your ability to fall asleep, especially since hypomania often disrupts the normal body clock that prepares you for sleep.

In their extreme form, racing thoughts are hard to miss. But milder forms may be more difficult to spot. One way of increasing your awareness of racing thoughts is to ask yourself some of the following questions when you are feeling energized or are shifting out of a depressed mood:

- "Have I been having more thoughts or finding it difficult to keep up with the pace of my thoughts?"
- "Am I finding it hard to focus, for example, am I having trouble reading more than a page or two, or watching a TV program?"
- "Am I having trouble participating in conversations because I move on to another idea before the other person is ready?"
- "Am I being drawn to things I wouldn't ordinarily notice? Do colors seem brighter, sounds fuller, smells richer?"
- "Do others seem slow or annoying?"
- "Is it hard to complete sentences or stay on one topic?"

Take the time now to outline what your experience of racing thoughts was like in the past.

What have racing (or quick) thoughts been like for you in the past at their lowest intensity?

_____

_____

_____

_____

_____

What have racing thoughts been like for you in the past at their highest intensity?

_____

_____

_____

_____

_____

MINDFULNESS STRATEGIES

Learning to pay mindful attention to the present moment can help de-escalate racing thoughts. Applying mindfulness to racing thoughts can help you slow down and promote a feeling of calm. Be aware that, in an energized state, you may have trouble doing these exercises for more than a couple of minutes at a time. Fortunately, repeated, short mindfulness activities can be very effective when you are too energized.

EXERCISE: MINDFUL BREATHING

One very useful practice is mindful breathing. Follow the steps below to practice this simple mindfulness exercise:

- Allow yourself to settle into a comfortable, seated position. Lower your glance a few feet in front of you or allow your eyes to close.
- As you settle, bring your attention to your breath. Breathe in for three seconds, counting one and two and three. Then hold the breath for four seconds (imagining pushing the breath to the bottom of your stomach). Finally, breathe out for five seconds, counting as you exhale.
- Repeat this for two to three minutes. Remember that your mind will wander, and when it does, gently return your attention to counting your breath.

EXERCISE: MINDFUL MUSIC LISTENING

Now try mindfully listening to music. Pick a song that's calming and familiar to you.

- Allow yourself to settle into a comfortable, seated position. Lower your glance a few feet in front of you or allow your eyes to close.
- As you settle, bring your attention to the lyrics of the song (if there are lyrics).
- After a minute or so of focusing your attention on the lyrics, allow your attention to shift to a specific instrument you can hear. Follow that instrument as the song progresses.
- Next, allow your attention to shift to a different instrument.
- Continue focusing on particular parts of the music for the remainder of the song, shifting from one instrument to the next, and gently bringing your attention back whenever your mind begins to wander.

A few other activities to consider trying are mindful coloring and mindful cooking. You could even mindfully wash the dishes! Any activity can be turned into a mindfulness exercise, if you are fully engaged with what you are doing in the present moment.

When you are practicing mindfulness, you naturally disengage from your racing thoughts and focus instead on the lived experience of the moment.

WHOLE-HEALTH STRATEGY

PROGRESSIVE MUSCLE RELAXATION

Research studies (for example, Chellew et al. 2015) have shown that this body-focused exercise supports physiological relaxation and reduces the levels of the stress hormone cortisol. Luckily, it's an easy exercise to learn, and all you need is a quiet place to sit or lie down for 10 to 15 minutes.

Focus on one area of your body at a time, starting with your toes and feet and working up to your head. Tense the area for five seconds and then relax the area for 10 seconds. Move through your entire body, allowing your full attention to focus on each specific area in turn.

- Feet and toes
- Legs
- Hips and buttocks

- Stomach and chest
- Back and shoulders
- Hands and fingers
- Arms
- Neck
- Mouth and jaw
- Forehead and eyes

Irritability and Agitation

Irritability and agitation are other symptoms that can occur when you are experiencing an energized or hypomanic state. Since hypomania is often associated with an improved mood, irritability and agitation can easily be missed.

The subjective experience of irritability is that the outside world has become particularly dumb or annoying. In other words, irritability isn't initially experienced as a change in mood. If you find yourself suddenly surrounded by the dumbest drivers in the world, you may want to consider the possibility that this reflects an increase in your own irritability rather than a sudden run of bad luck.

Agitation may feel like discomfort, distress, and unsettledness. For example, you may experience agitation as increased restlessness and fidgetiness. Often people describe feeling as if they can't sit still or focus. These symptoms can come on slowly or quickly and can last for brief or extended periods of time.

Irritability and agitation can have a profound effect on your relationships because they can lead to fights and arguments with friends or colleagues. It's very helpful to have a clear sense of how these symptoms manifest in your life so you can notice them early.

EXERCISE: BUILDING AWARENESS OF IRRITABILITY AND AGITATION

Below are some helpful questions to ask yourself if you think you might be experiencing an increase in irritability or agitation.

☐ Am I having more disagreements with people?

☐ Am I finding others more annoying?

☐ Am I feeling more easily frustrated?

☐ Am I being more assertive?

☐ Am I having more arguments?

☐ Am I threatening others?

☐ Am I getting into physical fights?

☐ Am I feeling more antsy or having difficulty sitting still? Have I been clenching my fists or wringing my hands?

Take some time to fill out the questions below to support yourself in gaining more awareness of how these symptoms have presented previously.

What have you noticed when you experienced irritability and agitation in the past?

_____

_____

_____

_____

How quickly did the symptoms come on? How long did they last?

_____

_____

_____

_____

MANAGEMENT STRATEGIES

Just as you used mindfulness and committed action to notice other hypomanic symptoms and create an action plan, there are practices you can use to increase your awareness of irritability and agitation. Use these exercises to examine ways to apply strategies that help increase awareness and reduce impulsive behavior.

EXERCISE: INCREASING AWARENESS

In the past, what thoughts or behaviors related to irritability and agitation have gotten in the way of your goals and values?

THOUGHTS	BEHAVIORS	CONSEQUENCES
"My coworker is an idiot."	I yelled at my coworker and called him names.	I got fired.

For example, if you catch yourself having the thought, "My colleague is an idiot," you may be inclined to respond by yelling; but if you reframe that statement with the more realistic, "My colleague made a mistake, but I still must work with him," you will be much less likely to say something provocative and unhelpful. Another option would be to think, "This is a thought I'm having because I'm irritable. What can I do to reduce this irritability?"

Strategies for relieving tension and stress reduce agitation and irritability. Examples include exercise, deep breathing, meditation, or removing yourself from a highly stimulating environment and spending time in a low-stimulus environment, such as a quiet or dark room.

It can be difficult to go directly from agitation to relaxation. Therefore, it can be useful to begin with a faster activity that is then slowed down. For example, try listening to fast music, then gradually move to slow music. Or, tense and relax your muscles through something called "progressive muscle relaxation" (see page 67).

Another important strategy to explore when you are coping with irritability and agitation is taking a break from conflict. You may want to pause an existing argument and resume the conversation later. You may want to take a break from people you are likely to get into arguments with. You might even want to take a day off work and contact your treatment team for additional support. We once had a patient who, when he noticed he was becoming most irritable, would take short camping and fishing trips away from home to avoid fights with his wife.

WHOLE-HEALTH STRATEGY

TRICKS FOR GETTING MORE SLEEP

Getting regular sleep is essential for managing your mood. If you are having trouble sleeping, here are a few tips:

- Keep your bed for sex and sleep only (avoid studying, watching TV, and so on).

- Avoid coffee, soda, chocolate, and energy drinks in the afternoon or altogether.

- Refrain from watching TV for 30 minutes before bedtime.

- Engage in a calming routine one hour prior to bedtime.

- Try not to eat heavy meals before bedtime.

- Do not use illuminated clocks.

- Try blue-blocking glasses (see page 58), which can be particularly helpful for preventing hypomania escalation.

EXERCISE:REFLECTING ON PAST EXPERIENCES

Take a few moments to think about your own experiences with irritability and agitation.

When this happened . . . :

I did this:

When this happened . . . :

I did this:

EXERCISE: IDENTIFYING HELPFUL TOOLS
AND PLANS FOR FUTURE USE

Was there anything in the past you found helpful in reducing irritability and agitation?

What strategies have you not tried that you would want to try in the future?

_____

_____

_____

_____

What are some things you can tell yourself in the future to disengage from conflict when you are more irritable and impulsive?

_____

_____

_____

_____

As with euphoria, grandiosity, and racing thoughts, when you start to notice an increase in irritability or agitation, make sure to prioritize sleep, practice calming activities, and avoid substances that can further elevate your mood. Reach out to your support system and care team as needed.

Takeaways and Next Steps

You should now be more aware of the various symptoms of hypomania—how they can affect you and how you can intervene earlier to prevent negative consequences.

Take the time now to go through the following checklist to review some additional symptoms and warning signs you may have experienced. Add examples and details where relevant to get as specific as possible. For example, if you experienced a decreased need for sleep, by how much did your sleep decrease? If you changed your appearance, provide specific examples, such as wearing brighter colors or not shaving. Consider asking a trusted friend or family member what signs they may have noticed in the past when you experienced hypomania, because sometimes those closest to you may have made observations you haven't.

☐ Decreased need for sleep

☐ Change in appetite

☐ Change of appearance

☐ Increased social media engagement

☐ Increased creative pursuits

☐ Increased interest in new hobbies or ideas

☐ Increased sex drive

☐ Increased spending

☐ Increased talkativeness

☐ Increase in other risky behaviors

Now write down three activities (for example, meditation, progressive muscle relaxation, mindful breathing) you will practice over the next two weeks to help when you experience these symptoms in the future (whether or not you are currently experiencing hypomanic symptoms).

_____

_____

_____

CHAPTER FIVE

Managing Depression: Dealing with Guilt, Hopelessness, & Sadness

IN THE PUBLIC MIND, MOOD DISORDERS are often associated with hypomania or mania, but you are probably more concerned about depression and its impact on your life—and with good reason. For most people with bipolar II, other bipolar, and cyclothymia, depression is the main challenge. This chapter discusses depression and its associated feelings, and gives you techniques to help manage them.

Depression is what causes the anguish that sometimes makes you feel hopeless. Depression is also what most affects your ability to function at work, at home, and in life.

In this chapter, we talk about effective techniques for counteracting depression's most troubling symptoms. Our work with hundreds of patients with bipolar has shown us that, when practiced consistently, these techniques can have a big positive influence.

Feelings of Hopelessness and Helplessness

SIGNS AND SYMPTOMS

Hopelessness is only mentioned in passing in the diagnostic criteria for major depression, and helplessness doesn't show up at all. Based on our experience, these two states of mind are central to the experience of chronic depression in bipolar.

Perhaps the problem with current descriptions of depressive symptoms is that they focus on single episodes rather than on the overall experience of a chronic condition like bipolar. Helplessness may not be a central feature of a single episode of depression, or two episodes spread out over 20 years, but over time, almost everybody who experiences repeated episodes of depression develops a sense of helplessness and hopelessness.

Someone trapped in the helplessness of chronic depression experiences the world as a series of threats to be avoided rather than as a set of challenges to be faced and overcome. There's a shift from a proactive approach to problems (trying to understand the problem and focusing on what one can do to resolve it) to a reactive approach (hiding from the problem and trying to avoid it). Repeated cycles of depression also lead to deep feelings of hopelessness, the fear that nothing will ever change.

Psychologist Jim McCullough has described chronic depression better than almost anybody else we know. In his view, helplessness is the loss of awareness of how what we do affects what happens to us.

Let's illustrate this with an example from our clinic. John is a 45-year-old business executive in Silicon Valley who has struggled for 30 years with the chronic depression associated with bipolar II. He works in a challenging environment and faces daily pressure to meet deadlines, but has been extremely successful in the past. Recently, his boss observed that he seemed to be struggling to meet expectations and drew him aside for a conversation.

John described the conversation during his next session in our clinic: "My boss has it in for me. Maybe he knows I have bipolar—I don't know. But I don't think there's anything I can do to change his mind. How will I be able to find another job now? I'm too old to look for work."

Listening to John, we found it easy to feel his sense of despair. We know that ageism is a very real feature of the tech industry, perhaps especially in Silicon Valley. And John has a family to support.

But then we remembered that something similar had happened 10 years before, also when John was depressed. That time, he was able to rally to overcome the challenges at work. First, he worked with us to understand exactly what his boss wanted from him that he wasn't delivering. In the process, he realized that he had been focusing on a project that wasn't important to his boss. He also realized that he had been sleeping in and showing up late for work, which certainly contributed to the perception that he wasn't doing his job. By focusing on those two areas, he was able to significantly improve his performance, and his next evaluation highlighted his success at handling the challenge.

We realized that the language his boss used both times was almost identical. The difference this time was that John seemed to have lost his awareness of how his behavior and willingness to take action could change things for the better. It was as though John's brain could no longer see the connection between his actions and his boss's response to him.

Before we could help him come up with a plan, we had to address the problem of his sense of helplessness.

MANAGING HELPLESSNESS

The first step in dealing with chronic helplessness is to recognize what's happening. If you identify with things we've touched on in our discussion of the psychology of helplessness, you're probably significantly affected by this problem. In fact, many of the seemingly unsolvable problems you face in relationships, at work, and in other parts of your life would probably be much more manageable if you could step out of reactive thinking.

This is easier said than done. You have been gradually sinking into the state of powerlessness over the course of the months, or even years, that you've been struggling with cyclical depression, so it's not likely you can change things overnight. But you can change things gradually. When you become aware of "hopeless" thinking as it occurs, you can evaluate it for things like accuracy and its helpfulness in your life.

You may want to carry around a notebook to track and practice the thought analysis exercise you tried in chapter 2 (Cognitive Restructuring, page 22) or explore phone apps where you can track and restructure these thoughts. Take a moment to decide which form of record keeping will work best for you.

Whenever you have experienced an emotionally challenging conversation (one that evokes negative emotions or feelings in you), jot down the answers to the questions in part 1 of the following Distressing Situation Review exercise as soon as you can. Within a week, do part 2 (Alternative Perspectives, page 79).

EXERCISE: DISTRESSING SITUATION REVIEW, PART 1—SUMMARY OF WHAT HAPPENED

Fill out this record right after a difficult conversation. It's essential that you write down exactly what the other person said as soon as possible after the event.

1. Date and time of the event:

2. Where were you?

3. What did the other person say to you that was most upsetting?
   (Try to remember their exact words.)

4. What was your gut-level reaction to what they said? What did you think they really meant by what they said?

5. How did you react to what they said? What did you say? (Try to remember your exact words.)

6. How did things turn out? Did you get what you wanted out of the conversation?

EXERCISE: DISTRESSING SITUATION REVIEW, PART 2—ALTERNATIVE PERSPECTIVES

Later, when you're no longer quite so upset about what happened, fill in this part.

What other possible meanings might you have taken from what the other person said?

1. _____

2. _____

3. _____

4. _____

How could the conversation have turned out differently if you hadn't interpreted the situation the way you did?

_____

_____

_____

Let's return to John to see how this kind of analysis is used in a real-life situation.

John had taken time off from work so he could visit his father on the other side of the country. John often feels that he doesn't matter to his father. As the two of them were waiting at baggage claim, his dad said, "Your brother is coming over for dinner. I think it's really great that he's willing to take time out from his busy schedule."

John's take on the situation was that his father was, once again, showing that what John does is unimportant. This is the gut-level reaction that he wrote on the form: "Great, I'm flying across the country to visit, and my dad just wants to talk about how wonderful my brother is for driving across town to join us for dinner. What's the point in trying?"

John answered his dad with a slightly sarcastic tone, "Yeah, that's just great." And then he sank into silence, fuming about his father's lack of appreciation. The rest of the trip was tense. By the end of his visit, John felt confirmed in his view that nothing he does matters.

Later, when John filled in the second part of the Distressing Situation Review, he found it hard to think of any other ways he might have perceived his father's comment.

This is typical when you first start doing this exercise. In the heat of your first reaction, it can be very hard to see alternatives to your interpretation.

However, John asked his wife to help him, and she said that if her father had made that comment when she was visiting, her reaction would have been quite different. She would have thought, "Wow, that's really nice that I'm going to be able to see my sister as well. Dad must want to have a special family dinner, since I'm visiting."

While John didn't think this was really what was going on in his situation, he was able to see how his view of the conversation affected the outcome of the visit with his father.

The next day, during a phone call, his dad once again commented how nice it was that his brother was able to join them for dinner during the visit. Having completed the exercise the day before, John was able to hold on to the awareness of alternative possible meanings. Instead of feeling sure that this was another example of his dad's thoughtlessness, he considered the possibility that what his father was really saying was that he enjoys it when the family can get together. This conversation ended better than his visit back home, and rather than feeling angry and resentful, John found himself remembering past family events that he enjoyed.

Feelings of Sadness and Worry

SIGNS AND SYMPTOMS

Feelings of sadness, emptiness, and sorrow are core symptoms of depression, sometimes accompanied by irritability and often associated with anxiety and worry. These feelings can trigger a profound sense that there's something very wrong, and this combination of emotions and the sense of foreboding can be one of the most disturbing aspects of depression.

In other words, it isn't just the emotion of sadness that afflicts us when we are depressed; it's the sense of something being profoundly wrong, or perhaps a feeling that something catastrophic is going to happen, that makes depression feel so unbearable. While it's natural to want to escape from these highly uncomfortable emotions, it turns out that many of the worst consequences of depression happen as a result of trying to avoid or escape those negative feelings.

Recently, psychotherapists have started focusing on taking the opposite approach. Rather than trying to avoid or escape from negative feelings, practicing mindfulness and acceptance therapies teaches us how to live with difficult feelings and carry on with our lives even as we experience them.

Several techniques from Acceptance and Commitment Therapy, which you're now familiar with from our work in previous chapters, can be helpful for people struggling with depression. The following exercise provides a way to practice these essential mental skills.

EXERCISE: ACCEPTANCE SELF-TALK

A key exercise that many people find helpful is to practice acceptance in their self-talk. In the early stages, this involves identifying the repetitive negative things we say to ourselves and, instead, trying out more positive ones. Practicing looking at painful emotions and thoughts in a different way can help us open up to present-moment awareness, cognitive defusion, and the acceptance of our negative emotions.

If you notice yourself having some "old thoughts," practice substituting "new thoughts." Using the filled-in items below as examples, generate alternatives to some of your own persistent negative thoughts.

OLD THOUGHT	NEW THOUGHT
I can't stand this depression.	It is unpleasant, but I can stand it.
It is not fair that I have to deal with this.	All of us must deal with painful emotions. Accepting this means not having to struggle with reality.
My life is ruined.	I am having the thought that my life is ruined. That thought is not "reality."
I must get away from this feeling.	I can find room for the feeling. And by creating that room, I don't have to struggle with it.

Lack of Energy

Three related sets of symptoms are common in depression: slow thoughts, speech, and movement; increased need for sleep; and a constant sense of fatigue or loss of energy.

Slowed thought and speech may be noticeable to other people. There may be pauses before answering even simple questions. And people who are depressed often move slowly as well.

Most people with bipolar depression experience an increased need for sleep when depressed (hypersomnia). Many people find it hard to wake up in the morning and become snooze-alarm addicts, lying in bed for an extra hour or two every morning.

However, when you're depressed, no amount of increased sleep prevents you from feeling tired. This is a situation when what your brain is saying you need is not accurate. Although you feel an overwhelming need to sleep, sleeping more when you're depressed actually tends to deepen your depression and lethargy.

HOW YOU FEEL WHEN YOU ARE DEPRESSED	THE TRUTH ABOUT DEPRESSION AND SLEEP
You feel you need to sleep late.	Waking up later in the day is one of the fastest ways to increase depression.
You feel you need more sleep.	Sleeping more than eight and a half hours a night is almost always associated with increased fatigue.
You feel you need a nap.	Naps that last more than an hour or so are likely to disrupt nighttime sleep and increase sleepiness.
You don't think you can do your usual morning exercise.	Skipping exercise for more than a day or two is more likely to make you tired.
Because you get up later, you have to rush to work; as a result, you don't get much light exposure in the morning.	Reduced light exposure leads to disrupted sleep patterns and more fatigue.

CREATE A SLEEP AND FATIGUE PLAN

Create a plan for coping effectively with fatigue and sleep changes that occur when you're depressed by choosing from these ideas and adding some of your own.

☐ **Buy or create for yourself a dawn simulator.** A dawn simulator gradually brightens your bedroom, which is a very effective way of helping you wake up in the morning, particularly in the fall and winter. Most of the devices you can buy are not bright enough, so look for a dawn simulator that can also function as a therapy light (maximum brightness of 10,000 lux). Or build one yourself by connecting lights that you can control through your Wi-Fi (for example, with Philips Hue lights) and a phone app that will gradually turn them on to full brightness.

☐ **Adjust your thermostat.** Your bedroom should be warmest in the morning, when you want to get out of bed. Bright light and a warm ambient temperature are much more effective "alarm clocks" than the typical ones that rely on sound.

☐ **Prepare for getting up in the morning.** Set out your clothes the night before. As you are going to sleep, tell yourself that when you wake up you will get right out of bed, put on your clothes, and get yourself a cup of coffee.

☐ **Buy blue-blocking glasses** (see page 58). Prepare for sleep by wearing them for the last couple of hours before bedtime.

☐ **Work your way back to eight hours of sleep.** If you have begun to sleep in, gradually change your wake-up time. Move the time you wake up by no more than one hour every five days so your internal clock has time to adapt to the change.

☐ **Work to strengthen your internal body clock.** If you have trouble with fatigue, get at least 30 minutes of bright light every morning. Buy a therapy light that provides 10,000 lux at one and a half feet. This will help you with depression as well as fatigue.

☐ **Get at least 30 minutes of activity a day.** The activity should raise your heart rate. Brisk walking is an excellent choice.

Trouble with Focus or Memory

SIGNS AND SYMPTOMS

Many people with depression have trouble thinking, concentrating, or even making minor decisions. They frequently grow concerned about memory difficulties and, if they are older, may believe they have suddenly developed symptoms of dementia. The cognitive impairment associated with depression can have devastating effects on a person's ability to function at work and in life.

Both anxiety and depression contribute to poor memory, although in different ways. Depression reduces the level of brain activity in critical areas of the brain involved in attention and memory. Anxiety, which is also linked to bipolar and cyclothymia, affects attention and memory; anxious thoughts take up brain capacity, reducing your ability to focus on tasks. Fortunately, there are techniques you can practice to improve your brain's ability to function.

MANAGEMENT STRATEGIES

Several activities can improve cognitive function in people with depression. Select activities from the following list that seem most useful.

- ☐ **Regular aerobic exercise** improves brain function.

- ☐ **Online brain exercise programs** have been shown to help cognitive functioning in people with bipolar and depression. You might want to try the Brain HQ program from Posit Science (see Resources on page 154).

- ☐ **Regular mindfulness practice** can reduce anxiety and improve the ability to focus attention.

- ☐ **The Mediterranean diet** has been associated with improved cognitive functioning.

NUTRITIONAL SUPPLEMENTS

If you're following the Mediterranean diet and you're getting outdoors regularly (to support your healthy circadian rhythms), you probably don't need any supplements.

If not, you might consider the following supplements:

- Fish oil (omega-3 fatty acids)

- Vitamin D3 (if you are deficient or don't go outdoors much)

- Methylfolate (if you have a genetic vulnerability to deficiency)

- B vitamins (if you don't get enough fruits and vegetables)

Negative Thoughts

Feelings of worthlessness and excessive or inappropriate guilt are examples of negative thoughts that commonly occur in people with depression.

These repetitive negative thoughts are examples of what are known as "automatic thoughts." Automatic thoughts occur without much, if any, conscious attention. In fact, they may be particularly likely to occur when the mind is drifting.

During a depression, we can become stuck in cycles of repetitive negative thoughts. We may regret the past or feel unlovable, or we may focus on all the negative things that could possibly happen in the future. These repetitive, automatic negative thoughts sap our motivation to actively solve problems.

What can you do?

MANAGEMENT STRATEGIES
EXERCISE: "TURNING TOWARD" THROUGH MINDFULNESS

Two general strategies seem to be most helpful.

1. Take back the resting brain from repetitive worry by practicing mindfulness meditation, which helps the resting brain disconnect from the parts of the brain that search for threats.

   One way of coping with negative thoughts using mindfulness is through an approach we call "turning toward." This involves noticing the thought that occurred, in addition to any sensations and emotions you experience when the thought arises. Instead of trying to escape or move away from the painful or uncomfortable thought, as we often do, practice observing your experience with curiosity.

   To do this, first become aware of when a negative thought occurs.

   What was the thought?

   _____

   Instead of trying to turn away from that thought, try turning toward it by noticing what physical sensations you experience when that thought comes up (warmth, pressure, heaviness, and so on). Where in your body do you feel those sensations? What size and shape do they take? Do they change when you observe them?

   _____

   _____

   Now put a name to the emotion(s) you experience when that thought and its accompanying sensations arise.

   _____

   _____

   Try practicing this a few times over the next week, when a negative thought arises. Give yourself a few minutes each time to observe your experience. How do the

THE BIPOLAR DISORDER WORKBOOK

sensations change? How do they stay the same? What do you notice when you turn toward instead of away?

_____

_____

_____

2. Activate the part of the brain that analyzes problems. This reduces automatic thinking. CBT techniques engage the parts of the brain that allow us to complete tasks, and as a result, suppress negative automatic thoughts. In other words, by actively analyzing the automatic negative thoughts, we replace that unhelpful rumination with real, goal-oriented thinking.

Thoughts of Death or Suicide

Thoughts of death or suicide are core symptoms of depression and, in some people, become extreme examples of negative automatic thoughts. Some of the people we have worked with have had periods of time when they thought of suicide more than anything else.

Reasons for thinking of suicide may include a wish to give up on what seems like a hopeless struggle against overwhelming challenges (financial, personal, emotional, and so on), a wish to end what seems like a state of anguish that may go on forever, an inability to imagine ever feeling joy in life, or the need to avoid being a burden to others. All these reasons usually contain serious flaws in logic or their underlying assumptions. One can always find a way to face or walk away from seemingly overwhelming challenges without killing oneself. No matter how deep the depression, it never goes on forever and is always followed by joyful periods.

Still, the logical flaws in these thoughts can be difficult to see. Some of the CBT techniques we've discussed and practiced in previous chapters may be useful. However, before turning to those techniques, you will find it's worth remembering that suicidal thoughts can become so compelling that no internal process will be able to change them. **It's essential that anyone who is experiencing suicidal thoughts has one or more people to whom they can talk about their feelings in an honest way.** This idea is discussed more fully elsewhere in the workbook (see page 10), but we repeat it here because relying only on personal resources to sort out a suicidal crisis is one part of what's wrong when people enter this state of mind. They forget their connections with others who care for them and, instead, feel that they must deal with overwhelming challenges alone.

Reminder: If you are currently feeling suicidal, call the National Suicide Prevention Lifeline at 1-800-273-8255. It's available 24 hours a day, seven days a week, and is free to anyone in the United States. Or turn to page 89 for information about steps to take right now.

Generally, most suicidal thoughts include three types of assumptions:

1. **Self-assumptions.** The person feels they are unworthy, unlovable, a failure, helpless, or fundamentally "broken." ("I'm worthless. People would be better off if I were gone. There's nothing I can do about it.")
2. **Assumptions about others.** The depressed person believes that others are rejecting, abusive, judgmental, or will abandon them. ("Nobody really cares about me; no one will ever love me.")
3. **Future assumptions.** The person with depression feels there is no hope for change. ("Things will never get better, and I can't tolerate feeling like this.")

All these assumptions are characterized by what is called "black-and-white thinking." Black-and-white thinking makes extreme judgments about the lack of any chance for positive change.

The state of mind that allows us to generate these kinds of thoughts is obviously not a calm and thoughtful state of mind. For that reason, interventions to prevent suicide must be simple and readily at hand.

A LIST OF REASONS TO LIVE

Make a business card–size list of reasons to live, and keep it in your wallet or purse. Choose from any of these that resonate with you, or make up ones for yourself, or get help from a friend.

☐ My faith

☐ Thoughts of suicide don't last, and then things seem better

☐ I might hurt myself and not die

☐ My family loves me

☐ My children need me

☐ I have a responsibility and commitment to a partner or spouse

☐ I have the courage to face life

☐ A special friend

☐ A pet

☐ My job

☐ Things I love to do

☐ Seeing my children grow up

☐ Meeting my grandchildren

☐ Helping others

☐ _____

☐ _____

ACTION PLAN FOR SUICIDAL THOUGHTS

Make another business card–size list of things to do when you have suicidal thoughts. Keep it in your pocket or purse.

- ☐ Go for a walk outside
- ☐ Do some exercise
- ☐ Play with a pet
- ☐ See a movie
- ☐ Watch a favorite film, YouTube clip, or TV show
- ☐ Listen to music
- ☐ Be creative (for example, draw, paint)
- ☐ Write something
- ☐ Get outdoors
- ☐ Do some gardening
- ☐ Practice relaxation techniques like breathing exercises, mindfulness, and meditation

- ☐ Take some time out to treat myself to a small thing I usually enjoy
- ☐ Take a shower or bath
- ☐ Go to a busy park
- ☐ Invite a friend over to watch a film
- ☐ Spend some time in a café
- ☐ Go to the library
- ☐ Go to a sports event
- ☐ Go to a concert or live show
- ☐ Talk to a special friend or family member: _____
- ☐ Call the National Suicide Prevention Lifeline: 1-800-273-8255
- ☐ Call my therapist or psychiatrist: _____

(Action plan from ReachOut Australia, www.au.reachout.com.)

Loss of Interest and Enjoyment (Anhedonia)

SIGNS AND SYMPTOMS

The loss of interest, pleasure, and enjoyment in life, called "anhedonia," is one of the central symptoms of depression. It may come on gradually and be so hard to notice that you aren't even aware of the change until you get no pleasure from doing something that's normally enjoyable and realize you haven't been getting pleasure out of any of the things you ordinarily enjoy doing.

One of the most effective self-help strategies for dealing with depression is called "behavioral activation" and refers to the process of doing healthy things that are or should be pleasurable.

Even if you don't get the normal amount of pleasure out of these activities, you will benefit from encouraging yourself to do one pleasurable activity a day. Gradually your ability to experience pleasure will increase.

Takeaways and Next Steps

In this chapter, we have covered a lot of ground. For most people with bipolar II, cyclothymia, and other bipolar disorders, depression is their most disturbing problem, so we have taken the time to cover these issues extensively.

To help you prioritize and remember the key points in this chapter, please rate the symptoms below from 1 to 7 in terms of their importance for you, with 1 meaning "most important" and 7 meaning "least important." Circle the one or two symptoms from the list below that are affecting you the most right now.

___ Chronic depression and feelings of hopelessness and helplessness; losing sight of your ability to make any changes in your life; approaching problems in a reactive rather than proactive way

___ Feelings of sadness and worry

___ Lack of energy or trouble with sleep

___ Problems with focus or memory

___ Negative thoughts and automatic negative thoughts

___ Suicidal thoughts

___ Loss of joy and pleasure

Now write down four activities you will practice over the next two weeks that will help with these symptoms (whether you are currently depressed or not).

_____

_____

_____

_____

_____

HEALTHY PLEASURES

From this list of pleasurable activities, choose ones you enjoy or used to enjoy, and create a set of healthy pleasures. Plan to do one activity per day for the next week and then check in with yourself to assess for positive impact on your overall mood.

☐ Doing something well at work

☐ Thinking of a future pleasure: a trip, a special dinner, a romantic night, and so on

☐ Expressing appreciation to someone

☐ Noticing beauty in nature

☐ Listening to a favorite piece of music

☐ Going to a museum

☐ Remembering pleasant times from childhood or the past

☐ Spending time with children or watching children play

☐ Participating in a group where you have a sense of community, perhaps a church or other organization

☐ Having a moment of silent meditation or prayer

☐ Putting your life in order

☐ Working well with others, or working as a volunteer on an important project

☐ Learning something interesting about the world, exploring an area you don't know enough about

☐ Going someplace you've never been in your hometown, playing the role of a tourist

☐ Going out for a good meal

☐ Seeing a special movie or play

☐ Watching a comedy special

☐ Shopping for a bargain

☐ Buying something sensual, such as perfume or bath salts

☐ Taking a bath

☐ Participating in a favorite sport or activity

☐ Gardening

☐ Knitting

☐ Cooking

☐ Playing a musical instrument

☐ Making art

☐ Touching someone you care about

☐ Sexual intimacy

☐ Romantic intimacy

☐ Learning to do something new, gaining new skills or knowledge

☐ Helping someone who needs help

☐ _____

☐ _____

☐ _____

☐ _____

☐ _____

CHAPTER SIX

Proceed with Caution: Managing High-Risk Behaviors

PEOPLE WITH BIPOLAR DISORDER OFTEN TEND to make impulsive and potentially risky decisions. Bipolar is associated with an approach to decision-making that focuses more on potential rewards than on possible risks. This tendency is present to some degree no matter what your mood, but it is considerably increased during energized or hypomanic episodes.

Hypomania and High-Risk Behaviors

A core symptom of hypomania is increased risk-taking. An overly optimistic sense of what is possible and an inability to see the risks in making certain choices can lead to impulsive decisions to spend beyond your means with activities like online shopping, going on a spending spree, buying a new car, gambling, and so on. A hypomanic or energized period is also a time when you might make unwise business investments based on overly optimistic assumptions; grandiosity can cause us to feel as if we're immune or untouchable.

Another core symptom of hypomania is increased socializing. If you combine increased social activity with increased risk-taking behavior, you may end up indulging in impulsive sexual encounters. You may choose inappropriate partners or forget to take normal precautions to prevent pregnancy and sexually transmitted disease. Or you might find yourself placing too much trust in strangers and getting into dangerous situations, like being out late at night in neighborhoods you'd ordinarily avoid or spending time with people who are doing other risky things, like using illegal drugs.

Another common example of risk-taking in hypomania is driving faster than usual. People who have been hypomanic almost always report that they drove faster and paid less attention to safe driving techniques when they were hypomanic, for example, by tailgating, speeding, or running red lights. Some people may even end up engaging in risky sports or sports they normally enjoy, but in an unsafe manner, for example, by skiing faster or in more dangerous terrain.

A particularly dangerous combination is the increased impulsivity and risk-taking behavior of hypomania combined with alcohol or drugs. The combination is very common: More than half of people with hypomania experience some episodes associated with alcohol or drug use (Cerullo and Strakowski 2007). Many people report *only* drinking heavily or using drugs when they are hypomanic and are, therefore, unable to see the risks of their behavior. And, of course, alcohol and drugs further reduce the awareness of risk and the ability to make thoughtful decisions. Because many of the catastrophic outcomes that can happen in a hypomanic or mixed hypomanic episode take place under the influence, it's especially important to establish ways of reducing access to alcohol or drugs during these times.

MIXED-STATE HIGH-RISK BEHAVIORS

As we have already seen, the dangers associated with bipolar are often due to combinations of increased energy and some other factor, for example, increased energy combined with alcohol or drug use.

One particularly dangerous combination is negative mood (pessimism or irritability) and increased energy, as we see in what are called "mixed episodes." Depending on the specific combination of the two mood states, we would either call it a "depressed state with mixed features" or a "hypomanic state with mixed features." The key, though, is the combination of negative mood and energy—and it can get you into trouble. A negative mood means the energy is often turned into potentially self-destructive activities. It is in mixed states that we see an increased risk of violent suicide and angry, self-destructive acts, as well as irritability and fights.

DEPRESSED HIGH-RISK BEHAVIORS

In a pure state of depression, the high-risk behaviors tend to be self-neglect or more passive forms of suicide, such as taking pills. The lack of ability to take care of basic needs can be especially problematic if the person with bipolar also has a medical problem (such as diabetes), where failure to care for oneself is potentially disastrous. Another serious concern involves bipolar parents or other bipolar people with dependents. While it's true that many parents do a better job of taking care of their children than themselves, it's also true that in a severe depression, it can become impossible even to care for your children.

EXERCISE: WHICH OF THESE HIGH-RISK BEHAVIORS HAVE YOU ENGAGED IN?

Check all that apply:

- ☐ Impulsive, unwise, or risky sexual relationships
- ☐ Spending money in ways that later caused you trouble
- ☐ Making risky business investments
- ☐ Trusting strangers too much and getting into dangerous situations
- ☐ Driving faster than usual and taking more risks
- ☐ Drinking or using drugs when hypomanic or energized
- ☐ Self-destructive or suicidal behaviors or plans for suicide
- ☐ Neglecting children or other dependents

Having a Plan

The key to successfully managing high-risk behaviors is having a plan. Taking the time right now to develop a crisis plan means you don't have to rely on other people to make decisions for you. Doing this ahead of time lets you think through past crises and the ways that worked the best to deal with them, which will lead to much better outcomes in the future.

Another important benefit of a crisis plan is that the process of developing the plan seems to reduce the risk of a crisis happening. Over our 20 years of treating people with bipolar, we have noticed that those who create a crisis plan before they do something potentially disruptive to mood stability (for example, taking a long trip abroad) rarely seem to need it. It's almost always those who didn't think through what they could do to prevent a crisis who get into trouble.

YOUR CRISIS PLAN

MY BASELINE

Go back to the exercise Find Your Baseline (page 51) and describe here your good, calm, baseline state.

_____

_____

_____

_____

MOOD PATTERNS

What have you learned about your usual mood patterns? Do you, for instance, tend to switch quickly from a depressed state into an energized one (hypomania) and then gradually come down into your baseline (depression-before-[hypo]mania, or "DMI"), or do you tend to switch quickly from hypomania into depression (burn out after being energized and crash into depression) and then gradually come out of the depression ([hypo]mania-before-depression, or "MDI")? Or do your moods follow another pattern?

My Typical Mood Sequence Is . . .

_____

_____

_____

_____

Mood Seasonal Patterns
Do your moods follow a seasonal pattern (for example, depression in the fall and hypomania in the spring, or vice versa)?

_____

_____

_____

_____

High-Risk Situations
Think back on the last few serious mood episodes. Were there particular triggers for these episodes (interpersonal conflict, substance use, high work stress, and so on)? Did they take place during travel?

_____

_____

_____

_____

Sleep Patterns

Are mood changes associated with changes in sleep? For example, do you shift into hypo-mania after a night or two of disrupted sleep? Or do you switch into depression after you sleep too much?

_____

_____

_____

_____

WARNING SIGNS

Other than changes in sleep, are there other early signs that your mood is shifting? One of our patients discovered that how often he posted on Twitter perfectly predicted shifts in mood: When he was getting hypomanic, his Twitter posts went way up. Early warning signs of hypomania might include having arguments with a spouse, drinking or using drugs, suddenly being more interested in sex, or spending somewhat more money. Warning signs of depression could include getting to work later than usual, having trouble answering e-mails, or avoiding listening to phone messages.

WARNING SIGNS OF HYPOMANIA

_____

_____

_____

_____

WARNING SIGNS OF A MIXED STATE

WARNING SIGNS OF DEPRESSION

THINGS THAT HELP

THINGS THAT HELP HYPOMANIA

You may have some specific activities that help bring you down when you are hypomanic. Examples include getting more sleep, doing calming and relaxing things, setting aside interesting projects, doing a short mindfulness exercise, and so on.

CIRCADIAN RHYTHM TOOL KIT

Healthy daily routines sustain healthy moods. Many people with bipolar have trouble regulating sleep, and as a result, their internal clocks (circadian rhythms) get out of alignment, resulting in poor sleep quality, daytime lethargy, and a greater vulnerability to mood episodes.

To sustain healthy circadian rhythms, you need the following:

* A way of getting up every morning. (We like using a dawn simulator to raise the lights in your room, although most dawn simulators are not bright enough.)

* A way of getting 30 minutes a day of bright light. (Direct sunlight is recommended, but how do you get it when commuting doesn't usually expose you to enough light?)

* An alternative source of bright light (10,000 lux at one and a half feet), usually a therapy light.

* A plan for getting daily social contact. If you work, this will occur naturally; if not, you might want to find some other morning social activity, like going to a coffee shop.

* A plan for regular exercise, which could include getting your 30 minutes of bright light.

* A way of avoiding late-night exposure to blue light (blue-blocking glasses).

* A nighttime routine for getting to sleep.

THINGS THAT HELP MIXED STATES

Usually the things that help hypomania also help with mixed states, but you may have some specific things you've learned work best for you.

_____

_____

_____

_____

THINGS THAT HELP DEPRESSION

What helps your depression? Many people find it helps to get out of bed earlier in the morning, restrict sleep to seven and a half hours, get more morning light, engage in regular physical activity, and talk to friends or family. This type of treatment is called chronotherapy.

_____

_____

_____

_____

Now you are ready to create your plan. Fill in the activities as appropriate in the table.

	MON	TUE	WED	THUR	FRI	SAT	SUN
Early Morning: Wake-Up Routine							
Early Morning: Light Exposure							
Morning: Social Contact							
Daytime: Exercise							
Evening: Light Avoidance							
Night: Bedtime Routine							

CRISIS PLANNING FOR DIFFERENT MOOD STATES

Think back on various times when you found yourself in crisis as a result of your bipolar II or cyclothymia symptoms, and you'll probably find that the type of crisis plans you needed depended on which mood you were experiencing: hypomania, a mixed state, or depression. Each mood state carries slightly different risks, so you should plan for potential crises with specific behaviors in mind.

For each type of crisis or risk-taking behavior below, describe the signs (behaviors) and symptoms (thoughts and feelings) that indicate you are in a crisis. Try to be as objective as possible. For example, "I am in a crisis when I get less than two hours' sleep for two nights in a row and don't recognize there's a problem" is clear and objective, but "I am in a crisis when I'm too manic" is not.

_____

_____

_____

_____

_____

_____

EXERCISE: WHEN I AM IN A CRISIS

CONTACT THESE PEOPLE

Family and Friends

_____

_____

_____

_____

Therapists and Doctors

_____

_____

_____

These Medications and Other Treatments Help

_____

_____

_____

SPECIFIC SITUATIONS

Risky Behavior with Money

If you have gotten into trouble spending money before, fill in this section.
Describe how you get into trouble with money. Do you shop online? Do you go out on shopping sprees? Do you gamble? Make investments?

_____

_____

_____

_____

Now describe the best way of helping you stay out of trouble. Write it this way: "When you think I am at risk with money, tell me this . . ."; "Offer to help in this way . . ."; "Remind me that these were my requests."

_____

_____

_____

Risky Behavior with Sex and Socializing

What kinds of risks do you get into that involve sex and socializing? Are you more likely to engage in unprotected sex, hang out with people who are sketchy, or take other risks?

_____

_____

_____

Now describe how someone can help you stay out of trouble. Write it this way: "When you think I am at risk with sex or socializing, tell me this . . ."; "Remind me to stay away from these kind of situations . . ."; "Offer to help in this way . . ."; "Remind me that these were my requests."

_____

_____

_____

Physical Danger

What kind of physical danger do you get into? Do you drive too fast or recklessly? Take risks in sports? Take other physical risks?

_____

_____

_____

Now describe how someone can help when you are putting yourself at physical risk. Write it this way: "When you think I am at risk . . . "; "Offer to keep my car keys or drive me somewhere . . ."; "Remind me that you are telling me this because I asked you to."

_____

_____

_____

_____

Risks Associated with Alcohol and Drug Use

What kind of alcohol or drug use is associated with being in a mood episode? Describe what substance you use and specifically why. For example, "When I am hypomanic, I use cocaine because I don't want the good mood to end." Then describe the negative consequence of that. For example, "When I use cocaine for too long, I get paranoid or crash even harder."

_____

_____

_____

_____

When you are at risk of alcohol or drug use, what do you want your support network to do? It is usually not a good idea to ask them to prevent you from using or drinking. It is often a good idea to have them encourage you to reach out to a source of support you have used in the past, perhaps a 12-step sponsor, a friend with similar problems, or a group that has helped in the past.

_____

_____

_____

_____

Deliberate Self-Harm

Suicide attempts and other ways that people in crisis may harm themselves (cutting, for example) tend to follow a pattern. Describe the types of self-harm you have previously thought of.

_____

_____

_____

_____

Reflect on the most serious period in the past. What were you thinking? For example, "I just wanted the pain to go away" or "I knew that if I cut myself, it would take my mind off these thoughts." And afterward, why were you glad you didn't kill yourself, or why did you regret hurting yourself?

_____

_____

_____

_____

What one thing would have helped you most in that moment? For example, "Telling someone how bad I felt and getting support," "Remembering that these bad thoughts only last for a few hours or days," "Being able to get to sleep." Describe the thing that would help you the most in those moments.

_____

_____

_____

_____

Whom should you contact? Whom do you most trust to confide in when you are in this kind of crisis?

_____

_____

_____

_____

RISK FROM NEGLECT

People with depression who need to care for others (children, for example), or people who have complicated medical problems or who are extremely depressed and unable to provide food, clothing, and shelter, may be at risk due to neglect. If this has ever been true for you, describe the type of problems you run into that threaten your well-being or that of others.

_____

_____

_____

_____

If you are depressed and unable to take care of your needs or the needs of those who depend on you, what kind of support do you need? Who could provide what you need?

_____

_____

_____

_____

WHEN YOU NEED MORE SUPPORT

If you are not getting well despite your best efforts, you may need more care. Regular outpatient care is sometimes not enough support. Here are some signs that you might need more intensive treatment:

- You have more than one problem that needs treatment. For example, you have a substance use problem and bipolar, or you have a medical condition that interferes with the treatment of your bipolar.

- You are having trouble taking care of your basic needs, or you are at risk of harming yourself or someone else because of your bipolar.

- You live in a chaotic and stressful environment that makes recovery extremely difficult.

- You have almost no sources of social support.

- You have a history of not responding to treatment in the past.

- You are extremely fearful of treatment and have trouble participating in your care.

- You are not sure you have a problem at all, even though everyone around you thinks you do.

If several of these statements apply to you, you may need more intensive care. Some or all of these options may be available in your community:

Intensive outpatient treatment. Seeing a therapist more than once a week, seeing a psychiatrist weekly, and participating in some groups.

Partial hospital program. Usually at least five to six hours every weekday of a combination of group and individual treatment. This is the most intensive nonresidential care.

Residential treatment. Generally a nonhospital setting where some staff are always around. During the day, you attend groups and individual treatment sessions, and at night, you stay in the treatment program. This is a voluntary treatment program.

Inpatient or hospital care. The most intensive treatment setting, this is usually the only place where involuntary treatment is provided to care for and provide constant supervision of people who are at risk of hurting themselves or others. It's also the best place to receive care if you have particularly complicated problems, especially if you have a mixture of medical and psychiatric conditions.

Capitalizing on Your Treatment Resources

It's important that you share this crisis plan with your therapist and doctor or psychiatrist. Get their input and suggestions. The plan must be yours, and it needs to reflect your priorities and values; but they may be able to give you a sense of what's realistic and likely to be effective.

You should also have a conversation with them about their availability after hours in a crisis, and when and how you should get in touch with them. If one of them is not available, whom should you contact? They should be able to give you answers.

Generally, your treatment team will be glad to hear from you when you reach out to them before you get into a full-blown crisis. Working with your treatment team to identify all the warning signs is one of the best ways of improving your quality of life.

Finally, see if your therapist and doctor or psychiatrist have any additional suggestions for treatments you have not tried. Several new treatments have been discovered in the last 10 years, including light and chronotherapy, transcranial magnetic stimulation (TMS), and other new medications and therapies.

Takeaways and Next Steps

This chapter has been a lot of hard work. If you have gone through it carefully and thoughtfully and filled out the exercises, you have taken the most important steps to prevent future crises.

If you would like to go further in developing a crisis plan, you may wish to consult the works of Mary Ellen Copeland. Her Wellness Recovery Action Plan was one of the first comprehensive approaches to creating a crisis plan and is the basis for her book, *The Depression Workbook.*

Be sure to share your crisis plan with close family and friends and with your treatment team. And make a note to update it at least once a year. Use the following next-step exercise to create a timeline for accomplishing these tasks.

ITEM	DATE FOR COMPLETION
I will have a finalized crisis plan by:	
I will share my crisis plan with my family and friends by:	
I will share my crisis plan with my treatment team by:	
I will update my crisis plan on:	

PART THREE

Don't Go It Alone

In this part of the workbook, we discuss ways to build your support system through your family, friends, treatment team, and community resources. You will learn more about how to foster healthy relationships through communication and problem-solving tools, in addition to examining ways to plan ahead with your loved ones how they can support you during times of both stability and crisis. You will also gain more information about the role psychiatrists, therapists, and support groups can play in supporting you to manage your symptoms and in promoting your overall well-being. Again, make copies of the exercises before filling them out in the work-book so you have some on hand for when you want to use them again.

CHAPTER SEVEN

Family Matters

ONE IMPORTANT WAY TO HELP MANAGE YOUR SYMPTOMS of bipolar II or cyclothymia is to consider how you can get your family and loved ones to provide you with the help you need, as part of your crisis plan and also extending beyond it. Having the support of those closest to you in identifying early warnings, applying helpful interventions, and promoting well-being can make a huge difference in your long-term wellness. It's important to think about whom you would like to include as part of your support system outside of your mental health treatment team. Incorporating family, whether chosen or biological, into your treatment plan can be very helpful, especially if you live with them. For others, loved ones such as friends and housemates can act as strong supports.

The people you want to include as supports may already be aware of your diagnosis; however, some may not be. Sharing information with others about your diagnosis is worth thinking through carefully. What information do you want to share, and what will the other person think you mean when you say, "I have bipolar"? Might they have misconceptions about what the diagnosis means? Will they have even heard of cyclothymia before? Also consider the best time and place to have a thoughtful conversation. Catching someone off guard while on the phone when they are at work is very different from sharing with them when the two of you are in a relaxed and private setting.

Sharing your diagnosis can help in many ways. It may increase your access to needed support. It may reduce your experience of stigma and shame and may enhance the connection you feel with others in your life. At the same time, sharing is a very personal choice and can leave you feeling vulnerable. If you have a therapist, it may help to talk through what information to share and with whom. Whatever your personal disclosure process, be sure you give careful thought to when, where, and with whom you want to discuss this sensitive matter.

Sharing can also create its own set of challenges. You may have already come across someone who responded to your self-disclosure in a frustrating or even hurtful way. Thinking through how you might cope with a less than ideal response reduces the potential negative effects of sharing.

Loved ones may be relieved to have a name for what you have been going through. However, bear in mind that they may have inaccurate information about bipolar disorder, especially bipolar II, cyclothymia, and other bipolar disorders. Providing educational information about these types of bipolar when you are discussing your diagnosis can help them clearly understand what you are saying.

In addition to exploring how to talk with your loved ones about bipolar and identifying how they can support you, this chapter will also help you improve your communication with loved ones and teach you some strategies for dealing with communication-related problems in family relationships.

Talking about Symptoms and Making Plans for Support

One of the reasons for talking with loved ones about your mood episodes, and the symptoms of those episodes, is to learn from one another. Each of us sees only a part of what happens. Even though you went through the episode, you may not have noticed everything that took place. And family members may misinterpret mood-related changes in your behavior. They may mistakenly attribute a very well-thought-out plan for starting a new business to a hypomanic episode.

The idea behind having family conversations is not to determine what "really" happened. All of us view experiences through the lens of our past experiences and our current mood. There is no undistorted reality. The goal is to acquire a fuller view of events by openly sharing our experiences.

It can also be important to identify ahead of time which warning signs you may be more open to hearing feedback about, versus others that might be less helpful or even create more conflict. For example, when you were depressed, your roommate noticed you slept later and showered less frequently. While hearing their concern about a change in your sleep might motivate you to apply some of the interventions you identified to avoid oversleeping, hearing their feedback about showering might increase feelings of shame and lead you to isolate more.

In the following exercises, take the opportunity to explore how and when you would want your loved ones to provide support. As always, a concrete plan created ahead of time is best.

ENERGIZED MOOD SYMPTOMS

EXERCISE: THINKING THROUGH A PLAN WITH YOUR FAMILY FOR DEALING WITH ENERGIZED MOOD SYMPTOMS

In the previous chapters, you created lists of early signs and symptoms of crises and were encouraged to share them with your loved ones. Take the time now to sit down with your loved ones and get as specific as possible to finalize your lists by going through the following questions:

Are there any signs and symptoms that should be added that have not already been included?

Is there anything on the list that is too constant to be helpful as a warning sign?

Is there anything on the list that would create conflict in a way that might make it unhelpful to include?

_____

_____

_____

_____

_____

Next, identify a plan for how and when you would like your family to intervene or offer support. You can do this by thinking through which interventions can be helpful when symptoms are just beginning and which interventions might be helpful when symptoms are high. The more collaborative you can be in this process, the more effective the plan will be. Together, think through some of the following questions:

- What do you see as a threshold for applying interventions?
- How does your loved one or family member feel about the threshold to intervene?
- Do they see other ideas for how to intervene when symptoms are high that you may not have included?
- How do you feel about those ideas?
- What would be good ways for them to express concern?
- What times do people express concerns around and what language can they use? Consider the language people can use and the time around expressing concern.
- What would be hardest to hear?

- What would be easiest?
- Is there any way they provided support in the past that you found especially helpful or unhelpful?

If you notice these early warning symptoms are occurring . . .

_____

_____

. . . you can provide support by . . .

_____

_____

If you notice these symptoms are high . . .

_____

_____

. . . you can provide support by . . .

_____

_____

If these symptoms are occurring . . .

_____

_____

. . . I would want you to reach out to the following treatment providers:

_____

_____

DEPRESSIVE SYMPTOMS

In the same way you worked through sharing about energized mood symptoms, it is also important to share and review depressive symptoms. What symptoms have your family seen in the past, and what are the best ways for them to provide you with support? As you share your list and add their observations, consider the questions you reviewed earlier.

EXERCISE: PLANNING FOR DEPRESSIVE MOOD SYMPTOMS WITH YOUR FAMILY

____ Are there any signs and symptoms that should be added that have not already been included?

____ Is there anything on the list that's too constant to be helpful?

____ Is there anything on the list that would create conflict in a way that might make it unhelpful to include?

Again, identify a plan for how and when you would like your loved ones to intervene or offer support. Bearing in mind your experience with depression, consider the following questions as you fill out the plan:

- What do you see as a threshold for applying interventions?
- How does your loved one or family member feel about the threshold to intervene?
- Do they see other ideas for how to intervene when symptoms are high that you may not have included?
- How do you feel about those ideas?
- What would be good ways for them to express concern?
- Consider the language people can use and the time around expressing concern.

- What would be hardest to hear?
- What would be easiest?
- Is there any way they provided support in the past that you found especially helpful or unhelpful?

If you notice these early warning symptoms are occurring, please help me by . . .

_____

_____

You can provide support by . . .

_____

_____

If these symptoms are occurring, please . . .

_____

_____

I would want you to reach out to these treatment providers:

_____

_____

PROMOTING HEALTH AND WELLNESS THROUGH YOUR SUPPORT NETWORK

Having a routine that promotes a healthy diet, sleep schedule, exercise, and regular engagement in positive activities supports your mood stability. Engaging your family and loved ones in related goals can be especially helpful in making the goals more readily achievable. Think through how you can involve your loved ones. Having an accountability buddy, or even a team, can help to reinforce your goals, especially when you are more depressed and your motivation might have decreased.

- Consider asking them to participate in your healthy activities, scheduling a weekly family walk, for example.

  Ideas:

  _____

  _____

  _____

- How could you involve them in creative, healthy meal preparation? Would you be interested in cooking together or trying new recipes?

  Ideas:

  _____

  _____

  _____

- Would you want to engage in exercise challenges or classes together on a regular basis? Perhaps you like going for weekend hikes or bike rides.

  Ideas:

  _____

  _____

  _____

- Could you create a weekly game night or a book club?

  Ideas:

  _____

  _____

  _____

Promoting Healthy Relationships

Relationships can influence your stress level, sleep patterns, or mood, so building healthy relationships with your loved ones through effective communication, problem-solving strategies, and perspective taking can further support you.

The skills we explore here can also support you in creating a space to process both your feelings and those of your family members with regard to past mood episodes. Close loved ones can experience their own pain as a result of watching someone they care for struggle with bipolar II or cyclothymia, as well as suffer the bad outcomes related to mood episodes. Financial effects, relationship indiscretions, or arguments that occurred in times of an energized or depressive mood state can all lead to feelings of anger, sadness, and disappointment. Additionally, your own anger or disappointment at how your loved ones managed a situation in the past, or guilt and shame you may be working through as a result of past episodes, can affect your relationships. Finding ways to talk with your loved ones can allow you to move forward and feel more connected, ultimately reinforcing your wellness.

COMMUNICATION SKILLS

Finding effective ways to communicate about grievances as they arise or process past disappointments can help you foster an environment with your family that supports your wellness.

EXERCISE: ACTIVE LISTENING

To begin, it's important to remember that a part of effective communication is learning how to listen and convey to the person you are communicating with that you are listening. While this may seem obvious, it can be difficult, especially during times of high conflict. Go through the checklist of key components of active listening to practice your active-listening skills. Which ones are you practicing now? Do you see any you know you need to work on?

☐ Maintain eye contact.

☐ Focus your attention on what they are saying to take in the information.

☐ Nod to indicate you are listening.

☐ Be aware of your posture and what it may convey.

☐ Ask clarifying questions as needed.

☐ Indicate your understanding of what they said by reflecting back what you heard, without adding judgment or criticism.

☐ Take the time near the end of the conversation to summarize what has been said, to demonstrate engagement, and to give the other person the chance to clarify if necessary.

EXERCISE: SHARING YOUR NEEDS AND FEELINGS

Talking about emotions such as disappointment, anger, or sadness is rarely easy, yet sharing feelings and being able to make requests for change is most often still worth doing. The tools below will help you practice this.

- Use "I" statements followed by facts, versus judgments. For example, "I felt angry when you didn't do the dishes after saying you would" versus "You still haven't done the dishes! You're lazy and don't care about me!" Imagine someone saying those different statements to you. Which one makes you want to follow up and do the dishes? How would each statement affect you differently?
- Remember to use a calm tone (not apologetic or loud, but firm and assertive).
- Request how you would like a situation to be handled differently in the future.

Use the space below to write out a few "I" statements and requests that you want to try out in the future.

_____

_____

_____

_____

_____

_____

_____

FAMILY THERAPY

Family therapy is an additional resource that can support you in managing your symptoms and promoting healthy relationships, ultimately reinforcing your well-being and overall health. In family therapy, you and your family meet with a third party (a therapist) to learn tools to enhance your relationships, and process and solve problems. Family-focused therapy can emphasize you and your family working together with a therapist to learn about aspects of bipolar and how to address symptoms and enhance support for you. It also works to highlight the ways family dynamics, conflict, and expression of emotions can work to either support or hinder wellness. With the support of a therapist, family therapy can offer you the opportunity to more deeply explore communication and problem-solving skills in order to decrease harsh expression of negative emotions (such as criticism or hostility) and to practice skills for listening actively, sharing feelings, and requesting change.

Jot down some topics you think would be helpful to discuss in family therapy.

1. _____

2. _____

3. _____

4. _____

5. _____

PROBLEM-SOLVING SKILLS

There have likely been times in the past when you made requests of loved ones that they didn't agree with or were not open to. That's where problem-solving can come in. These problem-solving strategies can help you come together with your loved ones to work out how to tackle a problem or find a compromise. Follow these steps to start a healthy problem-solving conversation with your loved ones.

1. **Identify the problem.** Begin by clearly defining the problem. Perhaps you don't initially agree on what the problem is. Taking the time up front to explore what the problem is will better equip you to tackle the next step of identifying possible solutions.

2. **Identify possible solutions.** Both you and your loved one should come up with as many possible solutions as you can. Write them down in a list.

3. **Weigh the pros and cons of different solutions.** What are the pros and cons of each identified solution on your list? Which ones best address the problem? Are there any solutions you agree on? If you cannot agree on one solution, is there a

compromise to be found, for example, trying out multiple solutions or trying out one person's idea this time and another's next time?

4. **Develop a plan to put the solution(s) you have chosen into action.** Outline the plan. Be as concrete as you can, including a timeline of when the plan will be put into action, if relevant.

5. **Revisit how the solution worked.** Schedule a time to check back in and see how the solution(s) worked. If a solution wasn't helpful, are there alternative solutions you could try?

EXERCISE: PROBLEM-SOLVING

Identify a recent problem that has come up between you and a loved one. Complete this exercise by using the space below to create a list of possible solutions along with their pros and cons.

The problem: _____

POSSIBLE SOLUTION	PROS	CONS

Action step: In the next week, I will (pick a solution from above) _____

_____

_____

We will revisit how well this solution worked on _____

_____

_____

EXERCISE: CONSIDERING OTHER PERSPECTIVES

When you are experiencing conflict or a disagreement where compromise is needed, considering the matter from another perspective can be extremely helpful in moving closer to reaching an accord. Try taking not only the perspective of the person you're in conflict with, but also that of a third party viewing things from the outside. This is an important interpersonal skill that can support deepening your empathy for others.

Think of the last time you were in conflict with a loved one.

- If you were to look at it from their perspective, what would you see?
- What about if you looked at it as a third-party viewer?
- What would you see on both sides?
- How might these different perspectives influence your approach to the situation?

Takeaways and Next Steps

In this chapter, you explored how to talk with your family and close loved ones about your disorder. You examined ways they can help you manage symptoms as they arise. You also explored ways to approach and address current conflict and process past challenges.

Knowing you are not alone in managing your illness can profoundly improve your well-being. In the next chapter, we will examine ways you can expand your support system outside of your family and loved ones.

Take a little time here, before moving on to the next chapter, to reflect on any current relationship conflicts that may be influencing your mood. Is there a way to use the skills you've learned in this chapter to find resolution? Use the space below to brainstorm.

CHAPTER EIGHT

Building a Support Network

BUILDING A SUPPORT NETWORK that includes a mental health treatment team and peers is an important aspect of managing bipolar II and cyclothymia. In this section, we take a closer look at medication management, therapy, and group support so you can learn in more detail what your support system could look like and how you can take steps to put those supports in place.

Medication Management

Medications aren't always part of the treatment plan for bipolar, but since they are a consideration, it's worth maintaining a relationship with a psychiatrist even if you are not currently taking medication. You may want to get together with such a consultant a couple of times a year. Of course, if medications are part of your treatment plan, you will want to get together more often, anywhere from once a week to once every couple of months.

Deciding if, or which, medications are right for you and making necessary changes in your medication depending on your symptoms can be crucial to managing bipolar II and cyclothymia. Finding a medication provider who's a good fit in your support network is therefore an important step. Usually, you can find a recommended provider through your insurance carrier or local clinic. Finding someone who specializes in mood disorders is especially helpful, although not always an available option. If you are connected with a support group or therapist, you can ask them for recommendations. If you have a therapist or will be seeking one, ideally look for one who can work with your medication provider, either in the same clinic or as part of coordinated care outside the clinic on a regular basis.

If you are taking medications, remember to communicate your concerns and any side effects. Your provider is there to help you explore your options and make changes when applicable. Stopping or changing a medication abruptly can have risks, so you will want to communicate with your health provider before taking any action. By speaking with them, you can ensure that any potential changes such as a dosage change, medication change, or ultimately discontinuing a medication, can be made using an approach that reduces potential risks.

You might find it useful to have a list of questions before meeting with your provider. Some questions to consider are the following:

- What are the potential side effects?
- How long do those side effects typically last?
- Are there any side effects I should follow up with you about immediately?
- How long does a specific medication typically take to see results?
- Are there any foods, substances, or other medications that may interact?
- What are the potential risks and benefits of the different medications?

EXERCISE: TALKING TO HEALTH CARE PROVIDERS

Take the time now to identify the questions you would like to ask a psychiatrist, physician, or psychotherapist. Also include any concerns you may want to discuss further:

_____

_____

_____

_____

_____

_____

It's important to check in with your medication provider about your diet in relationship to the medications you are taking. For example, if you are on lithium, it can be recommended that you not start a low-salt or salt-free diet suddenly. Make sure to follow up with your provider to ensure you are informed about any potential dietary recommendations.

Individual Therapy

Individual therapy is a great resource to support you in managing your moods. A therapist can help you come up with a monitoring system for symptoms and an intervention plan for if, or when, those symptoms occur. Individual therapy can also provide regular therapeutic tools that will help manage stress, relationship issues, or other symptoms, such as anxiety, all of which will inevitably affect your mood.

Therapy often means meeting with a psychologist, master-level therapist, counselor, or social worker weekly for about 50 minutes. The regularity and length of these sessions may vary depending on your symptoms throughout your time working with this person. It can be helpful to ask questions up front about a therapist's style, approach, and experience. Devoting time to finding someone who has specific experience working with bipolar spectrum disorders is important. Searching online, inquiring through your insurance provider, or asking for recommendations from trusted doctors or people in your community is another way of working toward finding someone who is a good fit.

Working with an individual therapist may not be a financial option for everyone, depending on cost, insurance coverage, and other considerations. Familiarize yourself with local resources, such as community support groups, workbooks, or online tools if therapy is not available to you. If you want to work with a therapist but are running into financial barriers, research local public clinics or therapists that offer a "sliding-scale" payment option

EXERCISE: RESEARCHING THERAPISTS

Take the time now to research local therapists based on the suggestions above. Identify three therapists you can call to learn more.

1. _____

2. _____

3. _____

EXERCISE: THINKING THROUGH QUESTIONS AHEAD OF TIME

Before reaching out to a therapist, create a list of questions. Some examples of helpful questions include:

- Do you have experience working with bipolar spectrum disorders?
- Do you use CBT or ACT strategies? How would you describe your therapeutic style?
- Do you work closely with any medication providers in the community?
- What are your fees, or do you offer a sliding scale or take insurance?

_____

_____

_____

_____

_____

We recommend sharing your daily mood chart (page 44) with your therapist and psychiatrist. This is an essential component of effective treatment, because it allows you and your team to monitor whether treatment is affecting your mood stability. Also, remember to share the crisis plan you created earlier (page 96) with all your providers.

Support Groups

It can be comforting to talk with others who have a diagnosis on the bipolar spectrum because they can relate to your ups and downs and the particular challenges you face. Having a place to voice your struggles and hear someone else say, "Me, too," or "This is what was helpful for me," can provide an additional and very helpful layer of support. Sharing about your challenges and accomplishments with a community of people who can relate to your experiences can also enhance your ability to stay well. Support groups offer a great space to build friendships and connections and can be a wonderful resource for recommendations of therapists or medication providers, relevant podcasts or blogs, helpful books, or even family resources for your loved ones.

You can often find groups through hospitals or local clinics. Using the Internet to do a search in your area can also be fruitful. Groups might range from peer support groups focused on mood disorders to psychoeducation and skill-building groups.

Peer support groups are led by individuals who identify as being part of that group. These groups are often free to join and vary based on location and who is in attendance. The Depression and Bipolar Support Alliance (DBSA) (see the Resources section, page 154) is a national resource that hosts peer-led groups around the country. Your local chapter may also be familiar with other resources in your area.

Hospitals and clinics may offer additional peer groups in addition to psychoeducation and skill-based groups. Psychoeducation groups focus on teaching you more about the disorder and ways to manage it, while also connecting you with others in the group who may be experiencing similar things. Other skill-based groups can teach you treatment approaches such as mindfulness or CBT. They offer another opportunity to connect with others while teaching you specific therapeutic skills. These groups are generally facilitated by a mental health provider.

While finding a support group specific to mood disorders can be especially helpful in expanding your network, groups outside this focus can also be valuable because having more people you feel connected to is foundational to enhancing wellness and managing stress. If mood-disorder support groups are not available, consider those organized by age (such as a young-adult group), gender, LGBT support groups, parent support groups, grief support groups, support groups related to a co-occurring medical condition, groups supporting those with co-occurring substance use (such as AA, SMART Recovery, Refuge Recovery, or LifeRing), or spiritual or religious groups you identify with.

Finding a support group that's a good fit can make all the difference. If you've tried one, it doesn't mean you've tried them all, since they can vary greatly from one to another. If you have an experience in one group that wasn't helpful, you may have a much better experience with another.

Going to a new group can be hard and, understandably, can create some anxiety. When thinking about trying out a new group, you may have some of those sticky thoughts, like "No one will like me," "This won't be helpful," and so on. These thoughts are common, so keep in mind that you are not alone. Don't forget to practice your CBT and ACT skills. You can also try weighing pros and cons.

EXERCISE: EXPLORING YOUR PROS AND CONS FOR SUPPORT GROUPS

Below is an opportunity for you to try the four-quadrant method: pros for going, pros for not going, cons for going, and cons for not going. While you may be familiar with the typical two-sided pros and cons list, the four-quadrant list allows you to dive even deeper into the decision-making process. As you will learn, sometimes the pros and cons for going differ from those for not going. By fully examining the reason for doing or not doing something, you can create a fuller picture of which decision is right for you. This exercise assists not only in fostering clarity, but also in building motivation.

PROS FOR ATTENDING	PROS FOR NOT ATTENDING
Example: "I'll meet new friends."	Example: "I will avoid feeling uncomfortable."

CONS FOR ATTENDING	CONS FOR NOT ATTENDING
Example: "It might not be helpful."	Example: "My parents will nag me."

FIND SUPPORT FOR YOUR FAMILY

Your overall well-being is tied to the well-being of those closest to you. In the midst of the ups and downs of bipolar and cyclothymia, it's sometimes easy to forget that your diagnosis also creates stress for those closest to you. NAMI, the National Alliance on Mental Illness, is a great resource and offers support groups for family members. Having support of their own through talking with other families who may be going through the same sorts of things and learning about ways of supporting you can really help your family members. NAMI local chapters tend to be knowledgeable about resources in your area. They may even have groups you can attend together. You can visit NAMI's website (www.Nami.org) to learn more about resources available online and closer to your home.

Use the space below to make a note of resources and groups, both online and local.

_____

_____

_____

_____

_____

_____

_____

_____

_____

In-person groups may be hard to access due to location and schedule, but you can also access groups online. DBSA, the resource discussed above, offers online peer support groups for people with mood disorders that can help you overcome potential location and transportation barriers. With today's advancing technology, online support groups are becoming more frequently available and can be found outside of DBSA. Take the time to search online to explore the best fit for you.

Takeaways and Next Steps

In this chapter, you learned more about expanding your support network through groups and treatment providers. Building these supports will assist you in managing stress, reinforcing wellness, and accessing help in times of need. Remember, if you use these methods of support but don't find improvement in your condition, consider accessing the additional levels of care discussed on page 108, such as intensive outpatient programs, partial hospitalization programs, residential treatment, or inpatient hospitalization.

It's important to recognize that asking for help from your support system can make you feel vulnerable. It's not always easy to share about the struggles you are going through or admit that at times, it's hard to do something on your own. Identifying specific people within your support system whom you trust and feel comfortable going to for different challenges can be especially valuable in overcoming barriers to asking for help.

It's also important to notice thoughts that can get in the way of reaching out to even these people at times. Thoughts such as "I don't want to be a bother," "They won't understand," or "I'm weak" can get in the way of asking for help. If these thoughts have come up for you in the past, know that they are very common.

Thoughts related to being a burden to others can be especially sticky. One thing that can help when challenging this particular line of thought is revisiting times when you helped someone else. What was that like for you? Were there times when you were happy to help or wanted to help? It's easy to forget that being in the role of helper can be very rewarding. As a helper, you can feel valued, respected, and maybe even honored that you were trusted enough to be asked. Try to remember this whenever you are feeling reluctant to reach out for help.

Explore some of these questions:

- What do you most want help with?
- What thoughts and feelings come up when you think of asking for help?
- What thoughts and feelings come up for you when you provide help to others?
- In what way can asking for help be in line with your values?
- How have you been successful in asking for help in the past?
- What was the outcome of asking for help in the past?
- How could you cope if you were disappointed by someone's response to your request for help?
- In which situations would you like to ask for help more often?

CHAPTER NINE

The Road Ahead: Checking In & Next Steps

YOU HAVE LEARNED MANY NEW SKILLS as you have worked your way through this book, and you're now much better prepared to cope, and live well, with your bipolar II or cyclothymia diagnosis. On the other hand, we have covered a lot of information in a short period of time, and you are almost certainly going to need more time to incorporate all this new information into your life.

Fortunately, you don't have to make all the changes at once; in fact, it's better to focus on a few skills at a time so that each of those skills is really mastered.

Take a moment here to review what was covered in the previous chapters and then prioritize your specific areas of concern as a first step toward developing a personalized plan for change.

Bipolar Types and Symptoms

In chapter 1, we started with an overview of the symptoms of bipolar and talked about some common misconceptions about the condition. You hopefully developed a clear sense of how your bipolar symptoms fit into the broad picture of symptoms other people with bipolar have experienced. The material in chapter 1 is worth rereading, but certain points are particularly important.

1. Although bipolar is defined by the presence of periods of increased energy (hypomania or mania), for most people, the most troubling symptom is depression.
2. To have a bipolar mood disorder, you need have had only one hypomanic or manic episode in your lifetime.
3. This workbook is focused on helping people with "softer" forms of bipolar: bipolar II, cyclothymia, and other bipolar disorder. It is not written for people with bipolar I, which is the diagnosis for people who have experienced at least one manic episode.
4. In addition to "pure" hypomanic and depressive episodes, many people experience mixtures of the two: mixed episodes.
5. Bipolar often occurs along with other symptoms. Of these, anxiety and substance use symptoms are the most common, and treatment for someone with bipolar often focuses on both mood symptoms and anxiety symptoms.

Review what you know now about your bipolar and what questions you may still have.

EXERCISE: DIAGNOSTIC CHECKLIST

What type of bipolar do you have?

☐ Cyclothymia   ☐ Other bipolar disorder

☐ Bipolar II   ☐ I'm not really sure

What other symptoms do you have along with bipolar?

☐ Social anxiety   ☐ Substance use

☐ PTSD (post-traumatic stress disorder)   ☐ Alcohol use

☐ Panic disorder   ☐ None of the above

☐ OCD (obsessive-compulsive disorder)   ☐ I'm not really sure

☐ Another type of anxiety

If you chose "I'm not really sure," don't worry—that can be a great starting point! The fact is that more problems occur when people jump to conclusions about bipolar than when they're comfortable with a bit of uncertainty and develop a plan to learn more.

Let's develop an action plan for learning more about your bipolar. Check any of the following items that appeal to you.

☐ I want to do some more reading.

At the end of this book is a list of Resources (page 154) for learning more about bipolar. If reading is a good way of getting answers for yourself, review the resources and choose a book to help you find out more about your bipolar.

☐ I want to keep track of my moods.

This is one of the best ways we know of to figure out the complicated pattern of mood changes over time in the relationship between mood and anxiety symptoms. In fact, making a commitment of just a minute or two a day to track your mood over time might be one of the most important things you can do to improve your mental health.

☐ I want to talk with a therapist or psychiatrist.

This is also an excellent next step, but make sure you're working with someone who knows about bipolar. At this point, you know a lot more about bipolar than many mental health professionals. If you want to avoid getting confused by contradictory information, find a mental health professional who is a bipolar expert.

Therapeutic Interventions

In chapter 2, you learned more about therapeutic interventions, and we discussed tools related to Cognitive Behavioral Therapy (CBT) and Acceptance and Commitment Therapy (ACT).

Here's a quick summary of the aspects of CBT that we explored:

- **The CBT triangle.** How your thoughts, feelings, and behaviors are interconnected (page 20).
- **Cognitive restructuring.** Learning how to identify when thoughts are inaccurate or unhelpful and how to come up with more balanced and helpful thoughts.
- **Behavioral activation.** How to use your behaviors to improve your symptoms and work toward your well-being.

You also learned how to apply techniques used in ACT.

Acceptance. Learning to accept the reality of what is, even when it's uncomfortable, can greatly reduce our pain and suffering and help us move forward.

Being present. Learning how to practice present-moment awareness intentionally and without judgment.

Values and committed action. Setting values-based goals and taking action that is aligned with your values.

Cognitive defusion. Coming to view your thoughts more objectively as temporary events, rather than as fixed external realities.

Of the specific exercises you practiced and topics you explored, which did you find the most useful, and why?

_____

_____

_____

_____

Remember, this workbook provides just an introduction to some of these techniques. Consider exploring these approaches further through other books and your own personal therapy.

Where Did You Start?

In chapter 3, we spent some time looking at your starting point in this voyage and how bipolar has affected your life up to now.

Let's summarize the information here. (Feel free to look over your answers and the other information in chapter 3 before responding.)

IMPACT OF BIPOLAR

Overall, how much has bipolar affected your life? Try to imagine what your life would look like at this point if you did not have bipolar. How much of a difference is there? Rate the impact as a percentage, with 0 percent meaning bipolar has had no effect on your life or an overall positive effect, 10 percent meaning a very slight negative effect, 25 percent meaning a significant negative effect, 50 percent meaning your quality of life is half what it would be without bipolar, 75 percent meaning you are hardly functioning at all compared with where you would be without bipolar, and 100 percent meaning impossible. (You would have to be dead.) Write your estimate here: _____

The purpose of this exercise is to gain a sense of how much you could potentially benefit from a program that helps you live well with bipolar.

Here is an example of how we use this exercise in our practice:

Robert is a man in his mid-30s who came to see us a few years ago. He was concerned that his bipolar was affecting his ability to succeed in his relationship and at work. He had held a series of jobs that started out well but ended after a few months, because he would fall into a depression. He was married, but his wife was very unhappy and, from time to time, talked about leaving him. In this exercise, he rated himself at 50 percent, but we suggested he might be closer to 25 percent worse off due to bipolar, since he was married and had been able to find jobs. In any event, we agreed there was a big impact from bipolar.

Then we looked at what he had done to deal with his bipolar. He had been to see a psychiatrist and had taken medications, but not always consistently. He had not done any kind of mood charting and had turned down the recommendation that he find a therapist. And he had done less reading about bipolar than his wife had. Overall, he had spent perhaps 10 hours (an average of 12 minutes a week) in the last year trying to deal with his bipolar.

Our conversation with Robert focused on this mismatch. He was a smart person who had seen a significant reduction in his quality of life, but he seemed to be reluctant to do much to improve his situation. It turned out he was very skeptical that anything he might do could help (see Feelings of Hopelessness and Helplessness, page 76).

So, we looked at that belief. It turned out that he got a significant benefit from the 10 hours he had spent. They had helped him resolve a crisis in his marriage and allowed him to hold on to his current job.

Through this process of analysis, we convinced Robert to increase his investment in self-care in a few strategic areas.

EXERCISE: HOW MUCH TIME HAVE YOU INVESTED IN BIPOLAR?

Thinking back on the past year (before you got this book), how much time per week did you invest in caring for your bipolar?

Seeing professionals: _____ hours per week

Doing homework: _____ hours per week

Other self-care: _____ hours per week

Mood charting: _____ hours per week

TOTAL: _____ hours per week

Now let's think about your situation. How would you assess your investment in bipolar compared to the impact bipolar has had on your life?

☐ I have put in lots of time. But I'm not sure it's paying off.

☐ I haven't put in much time. I'm just not sure it's worth it.

☐ I haven't put in that much time. I'm not sure why.

☐ I have put in plenty of time, and it's paying off.

If you checked the first box, that you aren't sure the time you have spent has been paying off, think through the lessons learned in this workbook. Are there some key areas where you put effort into things that didn't help? Write down your assessment of why those things didn't work out for you.

_____

_____

_____

_____

_____

If you haven't put in much time, but you have seen a significant negative impact on your life from bipolar, now is the time to commit some extra effort.

We often suggest starting off with a 2 percent investment. (We're pretty sure you think bipolar has had more than a 2 percent negative effect on your life.) That works out to about two hours a week.

Write down your commitment:

I am willing to invest _____ percent in improving my mental health.

In this same chapter, we also considered where you were in the process of recovery. Let's take a quick look at how your thinking and approach to bipolar has changed because of the work you've done in this workbook.

STAGES OF RECOVERY

Based on the Stages of Recovery model described on pages 46-47, what stage were you in when you started this workbook? How about now? Rate yourself before you started the workbook and now that you are approaching the end of it. Write "Then" and "Now" in the appropriate boxes for a quick visual summary of how far you've come.

STAGE	BEFORE STARTING THE WORKBOOK	AFTER FINISHING THE WORKBOOK
Pre-Contemplation "Others are concerned, but I'm not sure there's a problem."		
Contemplation "I need to do something, but I'm not quite ready."		
Planning "I am committed to change and making my plan."		
Active Phase: Crisis Resolution "Taking steps to get over a crisis"		
Active Phase: Building a Foundation "Getting all my symptoms under control"		
Active Phase: Living Well "Building a life worth living"		

We also reviewed developing a five-year plan, a process that can be very helpful in building motivation for change. Having in mind your goals for the future helps ensure that you make progress toward those goals.

Finally, we talked about the importance of setting up a daily mood chart. And we hope we convinced you to get started. This is one of the key points in our workbook and an activity that can make an enormous difference in long-term outcomes.

MANAGING HYPOMANIA

Part 2 of the workbook focused on managing hypomania and related symptoms. We talked about the importance of prioritizing sleep and normal daily rhythms (and about how blue-blocking glasses may help).

A daily pattern of activities serves as a powerful mood stabilizer. This routine should include between seven hours and eight and a half hours of sleep a night, preferably with a regular time of going to sleep and getting up. Healthy meals, regular exercise, and mindfulness meditation are also helpful. Many people find that filling in a weekly calendar helps them set up a routine that works for them.

We talked about the challenge of distinguishing between an energized mood and the normal relief anyone would feel when no longer depressed. Since an unrealistic sense of confidence (grandiosity) is a frequent symptom of hypomania, when you are in an energized state, it's wise to use a "48-hour rule" to prevent making unwise decisions. When considering any big decision, large purchase, or big lifestyle change, give yourself 48 hours to think it over before acting.

We also talked about how you can use the tools of mindfulness, defusion, and values-based committed action to help you avoid making mistakes when you are feeling energized or hypomanic.

Agitation and irritability are particularly disturbing symptoms of hypomanic and mixed states. It's important to realize that for most people, the experience of being irritable is a sense that everyone around you is suddenly behaving in an annoying or dumb way. In other words, most people don't initially experience irritability as a change in their own emotional state.

Irritability and grandiosity are emotional states that can lead to high-risk behaviors. But these behaviors can also happen in a depressed or mixed state.

Of the tools you learned in chapter 4 when exploring ways to manage hypomania, which are you planning to use?

☐ Prioritizing sleep

☐ Avoiding caffeine and other substances that can further destabilize your mood

☐ Engaging in calming activities (list at least three below)

_____

_____

☐ Creating a 48-hour rule before making important decisions

☐ Avoiding activities that may promote further excitement or conflict

☐ Using blue-blocking glasses

☐ Contacting your therapist or medication providers

☐ Restructuring thoughts

☐ Defusing thoughts

☐ Using mindfulness (list at least one exercise)

☐ Progressive muscle relaxation

In chapter 6 we discussed high-risk behaviors and how to avoid them. **The key is having a crisis plan.** One of the remarkable aspects of developing a crisis plan is that it seems to significantly reduce the risk that you will ever need it. In other words, just having a plan for what you will do and thinking through the circumstances that might lead to a crisis will help prevent you from getting into risky situations.

We strongly encourage you to fill in the crisis plan worksheet (page 96), or for a more complete version of a crisis plan, you can get an app for iPhone and Android called _WRAP_ (_Wellness Recovery Action Plan_). Either way, the time you take in developing this plan will be well worth it in the long run. And it will have a significant benefit on your relationships. Both friends and partners will appreciate the time you take to carefully create a crisis plan.

Sometimes we all need extra help, and we talk about situations that may lead to the need for more than just regular outpatient care. Intensive outpatient treatment or a partial hospital program may be just the thing to help you get through a particularly severe mood episode. For most of the people we see with bipolar, the biggest challenge is reaching out for help when it's needed.

COPING WITH DEPRESSION

Hypomania can certainly have a huge impact on a person's life, but for most folks with bipolar spectrum disorders, it is depression that's the number one problem. In chapter 5 we gave you several tools to help cope effectively with depressed moods.

We begin by talking about the impact of hopelessness on people who had repeated episodes of depression. The experience of recurrent or chronic depression changes our brains in ways that make it harder for us to see how we can regain control of our lives. A key change that takes place in how we face problems is a shift from proactive or problem-solving thinking to a reactive or avoidant approach.

If you've noticed that you're approaching problems in a different way or feeling less confident about your ability to make changes in your life, we strongly encourage you to use the Distressing Situation Review (page 78–79) to help understand and change this pattern.

One of the more challenging techniques to explain to people with depression is the notion that acceptance of negative emotions can *reduce* the unpleasantness of the emotions. Throughout this workbook, we have incorporated acceptance exercises, not because we want people to give up on changing their lives, but because change often begins when we stop avoiding the difficulties we face and instead accept our current situation.

Fatigue and sleep disturbance are significant problems for people with bipolar depression. We encourage you to spend some time regulating your sleep cycle using blue-blocking glasses when you are hypomanic, and a dawn simulator and a therapy light when you are depressed. Many of our patients find that using these techniques leads to a significant improvement in quality of life, energy, and mood stability.

All of us must deal with negative thoughts from time to time, but some of us can become mired in automatic negative thoughts. Sometimes mindfulness techniques can be helpful, while other people may find cognitive therapy tools, such as the automatic negative thought analysis (Cognitive Restructuring technique, page 22), more useful.

Thoughts of death or suicide can often consume us when we are depressed. The same state of mind that leads to suicidal thinking also tends to make us lose track of options and alternatives. For that reason, it can be literally lifesaving to carry around with you a list of reasons to live and an action plan for suicidal thoughts.

Life loses all flavor when we experience anhedonia (decreased interest and enjoyment) as the result of depression. We may have to force ourselves to do things that ordinarily would be enjoyable. The effort is often worth it, because this technique of forcing ourselves to do something we normally find pleasurable, known as "behavioral activation," is remarkably effective at reducing depression. Choose one healthy pleasure a day from the list on page 91, and you should notice a gradual reduction in your depression and anhedonia.

EXERCISE: COPING WITH DEPRESSION

When you are feeling depressed, it can be hard to do things you know would help you. For that reason, we asked you to create your own top depression strategies list (page 90). Go back and look at that list and update it as necessary. After you have reviewed the list, check the strategies from the following list that you have found most useful so far. Make a note, too, of which strategies you haven't tried yet but think might be useful in the future.

STRATEGY	TRIED WITH SUCCESS	WORTH CONSIDERING
Distressing Situation Analysis		
Acceptance Exercises		
Light and Darkness Regulation		
Automatic Negative Thought Analysis		
Suicidal Thoughts Plan		
Pleasurable Activities/Behavioral Activation		

FAMILY ISSUES

For most of us, family is important. But dealing with family when you have bipolar can be a challenge. Chapter 7 gives you some tools for addressing family concerns.

As we have already discussed, engaging your family in thinking through a crisis plan or plan for dealing with mood symptoms can change the nature of your family's involvement in your recovery. Everyone likes to know what they should do, and if you collaboratively come up with a plan for dealing with mood swings (making the plan when your mood is stable), it will reduce their anxiety and help them provide you with more support.

We also talk about some tools you can use to improve communication with your family. By using active listening techniques, you can better understand their perspective. And once you understand their perspective, assertive communication and problem-solving skills will help you express your own feelings and needs.

A support network usually includes more than just family members. You may want to have a psychiatrist or other prescribing clinician work with you. A therapist is often helpful as well. We talked about strategies for finding good therapists and psychiatrists in chapter 8. An important source of support can be other people who are dealing with bipolar, and we discussed various support groups that may be helpful in your recovery.

Go through this checklist, marking the items you have already completed that will assist you in building and promoting a healthy support system. Consider creating a plan to implement the items you have not yet checked!

☐ Incorporating your family's feedback into your symptom list

☐ Sharing your crisis plan with your family

☐ Sharing your crisis plan with your treatment team

☐ Practicing active-listening skills

☐ Looking at things from another perspective

☐ Practicing problem-solving

☐ Finding a psychiatrist

☐ Finding a therapist

☐ Finding a support group

Long-Term Outlook

Living with bipolar or cyclothymia is like a long-term relationship. It has its ups and downs, and problems we may have thought were resolved can come back in a different form. But if we look at it over the long term, we see that the effort we put into improving the relationship is well worth it.

For that reason, you will find it helpful to keep this workbook and consult it from time to time to revisit information and update the plans you've made based on your experiences.

It's prudent to anticipate that a major stressor such as a serious life challenge could cause symptoms to return. But you should also be confident in the knowledge that the work you put into your recovery from bipolar will increase your ability to master any future challenges.

TARGETING YOUR BIGGEST CHALLENGES

Think back to the five-year plan that you worked on in chapter 3 (page 52). What are some of the biggest challenges that you might face in reaching those goals?

_____

_____

_____

_____

What resources from this workbook can you use to overcome those challenges?

_____

_____

_____

What additional resources might you need?

☐ More information about _____

☐ Support from family or friends

☐ Help from a psychiatrist

☐ Help from a therapist

☐ Help from a support group or from other people with bipolar

FINDING WHAT WORKS FOR YOU

Let's take a moment to evaluate this program:

- Overall, what seems to have worked for you, and what hasn't been as helpful?
- Did you ever feel overwhelmed, or did you find that you were able to pace yourself as you went through the workbook?
- Did you get enough help? Too much?
- How often did you use the workbook? Daily? Weekly? From time to time?

Everybody needs to find their own sustainable pace.

"The thing I found most helpful about the workbook was . . ."

_____

_____

_____

_____

"The thing that was least helpful was . . ."

_____

_____

_____

Turn back to the beginning of this chapter and look at the How Much Time Have You Invested in Bipolar? exercise (page 142).

Given the effect of bipolar on your life (the importance of managing it well), how much time is reasonable for you to devote in the long term to coping well with your moods?

☐ _____ hours per day

☐ _____ hours per week

☐ _____ hours per month

Rate the activity areas below in order of priority (1 being your top priority) and then write down the specific activities you will do in each of the areas. Make sure your chosen activities will fit into the amount of time you feel you can commit.

My top activities for the future are . . .

___ Activities to improve my sleep and circadian rhythms

_____

_____

_____

___ Mood-monitoring activities

_____

_____

_____

___ Healthy-living activities

_____

_____

_____

___ Activities for coping with depression

_____

_____

_____

___ Activities for coping with hypomania

_____

_____

_____

A FINAL WORD

CONGRATULATIONS! You have made your way through this workbook and learned many new skills to manage your bipolar II or cyclothymia. Living well with bipolar can be challenging, but our experience working with many people with bipolar in our practice has shown us that success is absolutely possible. All the time and effort you have put into completing this workbook will pay off in many rewarding ways over the next few years. With your new skills and increased knowledge of bipolar, you will find your own path (with your support network, of course!) to living well. People with bipolar have demonstrated again and again their creativity in finding new strategies for coping with their challenges, and we truly believe you will, too. Here's to your success!

RESOURCES

WEBSITES

BrainHQ provides apps for research-based exercises to improve cognitive health in various ways. www.brainhq.com

Depression and Bipolar Support Alliance (DBSA) has resources and support groups for people with bipolar. www.dbsalliance.org

Our clinic, **Gateway Psychiatric Services**, has a website with lots of information about bipolar and other mood disorders. www.gatewaypsychiatric.com

Mood Surfing has many resources specific to the treatment and management of mood disorders. www.moodsurfing.com

The National Alliance on Mental Illness (NAMI) has useful resources and support groups for people struggling with many different mental disorders and for their family members. www.nami.org

Dr. Jim Phelps's **PsychEducation** website has information about medications and mood symptoms associated with the bipolar spectrum. www.psycheducation.org

Psychology Tools is a site offering many helpful bipolar tools, including treatment guides, CBT worksheets, and more. www.psychologytools.com/bipolar.html

FURTHER READING

ACT RESOURCES

ACT Made Simple: An Easy-To-Read Primer on Acceptance and Commitment Therapy by Russ Harris. Oakland, CA: New Harbinger Publications (2009).

Get Out of Your Mind and Into Your Life: The New Acceptance and Commitment Therapy by Steven Hayes. Oakland, CA: New Harbinger Publications (2005).

CBT RESOURCES

The Bipolar Workbook: Tools for Controlling Your Mood Swings (2nd ed.) by Monica Ramirez Basco. New York: Guilford Press (2015).

Managing Bipolar Disorder: A Cognitive Behavior Treatment Program Workbook by Michael W. Otto, Noreen A. Reilly-Harrington, Jane N. Kogan, Aude Hein, Robert O. Knauz, and Gary S. Sachs. New York: Oxford University Press (2009).

PTSD AND ANXIETY RESOURCES

Acceptance and Commitment Therapy for Anxiety Disorders: A Practitioner's Treatment Guide to Using Mindfulness, Acceptance, and Values-Based Behavior Change Strategies by Georg H. Eifert and John P. Forsyth. Oakland: New Harbinger Publications (2005).

Birth of a New Brain: Healing from Postpartum Bipolar Disorder by Dyane Harwood. New York: Post Hill Press (2017).

Mastery of Your Anxiety and Panic: Workbook for Primary Care Settings by Michelle G. Craske and David H. Barlow. New York: Oxford University Press (2007).

Reclaiming Your Life from a Traumatic Experience Workbook by Barbara Olasov Rothbaum, Edna B. Foa, and Elizabeth A. Hembree. New York: Oxford University Press (2007).

REFERENCES

Barnett, J. H., and J. W. Smoller. "The Genetics of Bipolar Disorder." *Neuroscience* 164, no. 1 (2009): 331–43. doi:10.1016/j.neuroscience.2009.03.080.

Cerullo, M. A., and S. M. Strakowski. "The Prevalence and Significance of Substance Use Disorders in Bipolar Type I and II Disorder." *Substance Abuse Treatment, Prevention, and Policy* 2 (October 2007): 29. doi:10.1186/1747-597X-2-29.

Chellew, K., P. Evans, J. Fornes-Vives, G. Pérez, and G. Garcia-Banda. "The Effect of Progressive Muscle Relaxation on Daily Cortisol Secretion." *Stress* 18, no. 5 (2015): 538–44. doi:10.3109/10253890.2015.1053454.

Copeland, Mary Ellen. *Wellness Recovery Action Plan (WRAP)*. Brookline Village, MA: Mental Illness Education Project Inc., 2002.

Davidson, R. J., J. Kabat-Zinn, J. Schumacher, M. Rosenkranz, D. Muller, S. F. Santorelli, F. Urbanowski, A. Harrington, K. Bonus, and J. F. Sheridan. "Alterations in Brain and Immune Function Produced by Mindfulness Meditation." *Psychosomatic Medicine* 65, no. 4 (2003): 564–70.

Frank, Ellen. *Treating Bipolar Disorder: A Clinician's Guide to Interpersonal and Social Rhythm Therapy*. New York: Guilford Press, 2005.

Gartner, John D. *The Hypomanic Edge: The Link between (a Little) Craziness and (a Lot of) Success in America*. New York: Simon & Schuster, 2011.

Hamilton, J. P., M. Farmer, P. Fogelman, and I. H. Gotlib. "Depressive Rumination, the Default-Mode Network, and the Dark Matter of Clinical Neuroscience." *Biological Psychiatry* 78, no. 4 (2015): 224–30.

Hayes, Steven C., Kirk D. Strosahl, and Kelly G. Wilson. *Acceptance and Commitment Therapy: An Experiential Approach to Behavior Change*. New York: Guilford Press, 1999.

Henriksen T. E., S. Skrede, O. B. Fasmer, H. Schoeyen, I. Leskauskaite, J. Bjørke-Bertheussen, J. Assmus, B. Hamre, J. Grønli, and A. Lund. "Blue-Blocking Glasses as Additive Treatment for Mania: A Randomized Placebo-Controlled Trial." *Bipolar Disorder* 18, no. 3 (2016): 221–32.

Jamison, Kay Redfield. *Touched with Fire: Manic-Depressive Illness and the Artistic Temperament*. New York: Free Press, 1996.

Kabat-Zinn, Jon. *Wherever You Go, There You Are: Mindfulness Meditation in Everyday Life*. New York: Hyperion, 1994.

McCullough Jr., James P. *Treatment for Chronic Depression: Cognitive Behavioral Analysis System of Psychotherapy (CBASP)*. New York: Guilford Press, 2000.

Parletta, N., D. Zarnowiecki, J. Cho, A. Wilson, S. Bogomolova, A. Villani, C. Itsiopoulos, T. Niyonsenga, S. Blunden, B. Meyer, L. Segal, B. T. Baune, and K. O'Dea. "A Mediterranean-Style Dietary Intervention Supplemented with Fish Oil Improves Diet Quality and Mental Health in People with Depression: A Randomized Controlled Trial (HELFIMED)." *Nutritional Neuroscience* 7 (December 2017): 1–14. doi:10.1080/1028415X.2017.1411320.

Prochaska, James O., and Carlo C. DiClemente. *The Transtheoretical Approach: Crossing Traditional Boundaries of Therapy*. Homewood, IL: Dow Jones-Irwin, 1984.

Rogers, Carl R. *On Becoming a Person: A Therapist's View of Psychotherapy*. 2nd ed. New York: Houghton Mifflin, 1995.

Üstün, T. B., N. Kostanjsek, and S. Chatterji, eds. *Measuring Health and Disability: Manual for WHO Disability Assessment Schedule (WHODAS 2.0)*. Geneva: World Health Organization, 2010.

Zagorski, N. "Blue Light–Blocking Glasses May Reduce Bipolar Mania." *Psychiatric News* online ed., August 18, 2016. https://doi.org/10.1176/appi.pn.2016.8a24.

INDEX

ABOUT THE AUTHORS

DR. FORSTER is a clinical professor of psychiatry at the University of California, San Francisco, where he teaches on the diagnosis and treatment of bipolar disorder and supervises the psychiatry residents in the Bipolar Clinic. He is also clinical director of Gateway Psychiatric Services, a multidisciplinary clinic focused on combining medication and psychotherapy in the treatment of people with recurrent mood disorders. He is a distinguished fellow of the American Psychiatric Association and the author of many academic works on the treatment and diagnosis of bipolar disorder, among other topics. He has been an invited speaker at conferences around the United States and in Asia and Europe.

GINA GREGORY is a licensed clinical social worker who earned her degree from the University of California, Berkeley, with a concentration in community mental health. She first began working with individuals with mood disorders during graduate school in 2011. She has worked at an early-intervention clinic for individuals recently diagnosed with bipolar disorder and at a dual-diagnosis clinic serving adults with substance use and mood disorders, and she continues to serve individuals with mood disorders at Gateway Psychiatric Services. She is committed to supporting people with mood disorders and their families in accessing and developing resources to help them manage symptoms and work toward wellness.